The British Aestheticians Guide To

Waxing The Twigs & Berries

Claire Barnes

authorHOUSE®

AuthorHouse™
1663 Liberty Drive
Bloomington, IN 47403
www.authorhouse.com
Phone: 1-800-839-8640

First published by AuthorHouse−09/08/2011

ISBN: 978-1-4634-3275-1 (sc)
ISBN: 978-1-4634-3460-1 (ebk)

Library of Congress Control Number: 2011911528

Printed in the United States of America

Cover Design by Carolyn Sheltraw, www.csheltraw.com

Contents

Acknowledgements

I would like to thank Carolyn Sheltraw, Amy Honaker, Drew Ferraro and Jara Harris for all participating in some way towards the development of this book.

I would also love to give a big 'thanks' to all who participated in the "Real Life" chapter of this book.

And, not to forget Nina Gass, my wonderful editor who I don't think has ever had to edit a book with such terms as scrotum, twigs, and berries before! Cheers!

There are many things I have been called in my life, but the one name that I cherish the most is "Mum"—so on that note I would love to thank last but not least my two children, Dylan and Penny, for their patience whilst I got my knickers in a twist from time to time, juggling my life and trying to write this book. Love you dearly, thank you!

You are all truly wonderful and, without you, my book would not be complete!

Preface

To all my lovely professional readers who are licensed, or about to be licensed in the aesthetics trade, this isn't intended as your only training tool but one that should supplement DVDs and hands-on training classes with professionals already in the know before you let yourself loose on a paying client. Round up your friends and your existing clients, give out free guinea pig waxing sessions, and be sure to get your technique up to high expectations before you charge your clients. Along the way, this guide is here to provide some tid-bits of valuable information that you maybe didn't pick up in beauty school or in other areas of training once you became licensed. Also, please check that the state that you are licensed in is in acceptance of the services that you offer in your salon. All states within the U.S.A have their own rules and regulations when it comes to waxing.

The content of this manual is meant to be informative in a fun and cheeky way and is focused primarily on waxing the male nether regions. After attending different waxing classes and talking with lots of other professionals so that I could learn what to do and what not to do and watching DVDs, coupled with hands-on waxing of male body parts over the years, I learnt very quickly what worked best for me. Essentially, I found that the application and removal of wax is no different to that of waxing the female nether regions and is not just limited to the sacred areas spoken of in this book. So, please by all means, take this knowledge of wax and its wonderful capabilities with you to all areas of the male/female body throughout your waxing profession.

Some of the content written in the book isn't intended to offend anybody and, hence, why I have resorted to certain euphemisms. I am hoping it makes you snigger just a little bit and makes you feel more confident about this service and about the male anatomy when it comes to waxing. For any of you not familiar with some of the British phrases, there is a glossary at the end of this book to "translate" my meaning.

I hope that any of the descriptive terms used to describe the guy's intimate body parts don't offend anybody. If they do, maybe this book isn't the best match for you or just maybe you want to use medical terms to describe their parts. Whatever the case, all are fine, and I am not twisting your arm, or threatening you that you must continue reading this manual.

Thank you for reading!

All things are difficult before they are easy.
Thomas Fuller

What are the Twigs and Berries?

Quite simply, this is a cheeky, fun term that is often used in England to describe the male body parts located downstairs. In this manual, you may find that I use other typical British terminology to also describe them, but Twigs and Berries are my favourite term—hence the title of my book.

In a nutshell, the twigs (even though your client might not resemble a twig) are what we shall refer to as the male private body parts—the lunch box, his manhood, penis or whatever term you like to use.

I was once asked by a much younger aesthetician, "What is the difference between the testes and the scrotum?" The testes basically are the wobbly bits that are held in place by the sack (also known as the scrotum). With my clients, I tend to use the term, scrotum, as it is the scrotum skin that we are protecting and working on and not really the testes. Hope this makes sense.

Men tend to dislike body hair down there just as much as women. It is all personal preference. It is becoming increasingly popular though and more and more men are starting to look into having this done.

Some men say, "It actually makes the junk look bigger" Hey? What man do you know, that wouldn't mind that? They also report back to me that when their partner has a waxing down there also, it increases their sexual satisfaction and makes for a better sex life. It's a great selling tool (excuse the pun) to ask your male clients if they want to increase their sex life and you can show them how!! Cha-ching!

What Can He Expect When
Getting His Waxing Service?

Don't expect him to take a nap during this service. If taking the occasional phone call during the service is what floats his boat and if the person on the other end of the phone is okay with some slight heavy breathing, gasps of breath or mutterings of obscenities down the other end of the phone, then tell your client to go ahead. Personally, it would be easier if your client cooperated with you as he is there to help assist with keeping his skin taut for you and you will need both of his hands. If he can chat on the phone, hands free then tell him to go for it!

Your client should expect some discomfort, especially if it is his first time being waxed, and especially if it is his first time having a "Manzilian." He should expect to work for his service by holding himself at times to allow you to apply the wax and remove it. He will need to stretch his skin to assist you in the process and bend his legs from time to time so that you can get into those nooks and safely remove the wax without hurting him or bruising him.

Most clients tell me that the most painful part of the "Manzilian" is the top part around his twig where the hair is denser. The scrotum, they tell me, really doesn't hurt that much, but when I think about waxing a female, most females say the same thing. Well, they don't have a scrotum, but the labia, doesn't hurt as much as their pubic bone area does.

The scrotum is very thin, so you have to be EXTREMELY careful when waxing this area. Time and consideration must be taken into account and the type of wax you use is also crucial when waxing this area. Waxing this area is where you will require the most help from him. At all times when applying the wax around the scrotum and removing it, you will need his assistance with stretching and pulling the skin taut to aid in the process.

He will love the results and, once you get him hooked, there will be no going back. He may feel a bit tender for a few hours after he has had his waxing and even a bit of itching is to be expected. Send him home with a good soothing cream (I recommend a good one for him to use later on in the book) and tell him to ask his partner to rub the lotion in to soothe the delicate spots. Call it bonding time!

The Questionnaire

First, you will need to ask him to fill out a questionnaire. (Boring I know as most people hate it when they are handed those pesky things to fill in, and some of the questions seem to be completely irrelevant to the service or visit that they are participating in.) You know the ones with endless questions regarding what medications they are on, etc.

Acutane and Retin-A: If the client is using any of these lotions/medications for acne or fine lines, you will need to tell him to hold off on waxing for two weeks since he last applied the Retin-A and at least six months since he last used Acutane.

These products cause thinning of the skin as they are both Keratolytics. Keratolytics increase the speed of skin exfoliation and, even though they may use this product on the face for acne or fine lines—and not necessarily around "the berries"—the product 'migrates' which means it gets into the blood stream through the pores and just causes a whole array of problems when combined with waxing. Typically, when clients use these products and have a wax, the skin due to its sensitivity will burn. Sometimes the scars from the wax burn can also be permanent.

You will also have to ask him if he suffers from herpes or any other sexually transmitted disease (STD). This isn't because we are nosey; we just want to protect ourselves and, more importantly, if your client is susceptible to these diseases, we don't want to spread it or bring on those little herpes buggers that might be lying dormant!

Your questionnaire should also consist of questions about whether they are on blood thinners, whether they are vitamin deficient, or if they take aspirin daily. Knowing the answers to these questions helps you to be more aware of their potential to bruising.

Another question I think is important to ask is if they have a pacemaker or if they are epileptic. I go into why I ask this question in Tip 11 on high frequency later in the book.

Some of the questions do seem boring and pointless, but it is very important that we know the answers before any waxing service. From waxing eyebrows to the hairs on their toes, we need to understand what medications they are taking before we go ahead.

When he has filled out the form, be sure to then read it. Don't just take it for granted that he is Mr. Clean Bill of Health. With any answers that he gives to you, spend some time with him and discuss any concerns or further questions that you may have.

You also need to inform your clients why you are asking these questions. There is nothing wrong with telling a client that using Retin-A when waxing can cause him/her to lose half their skin due to increased exfoliation of the skin brought on by that medication. Unless the client is a real cheeky monkey, then they should understand why it is important to be honest—otherwise, they will pay the consequences.

We all have our little secrets, and, over the years, I have found that it is more likely to be a female client that tells little fibs about her use of Retin-A. Maybe they want people to think their flawless complexion and wrinkle-free face is all down to natural perfection, so they withhold from sharing this information. It is all good, but once you have explained to the client the reasoning behind your questions, we would hope that they would then fess up!

The number 'one' reason why salons or spa's are sued in the U.S.A is from 'waxing'! Protect yourselves and do not be complacent with your client's safety. It might come back to bite you in the bum!

The next chapter covers all contraindications for waxing in general. Please read it as it is important that you know these things and have these questions on your questionnaire form.

Contraindications to All Waxing

Some doctors do not recommend waxing for people who are diabetic, have poor circulation or who have varicose veins. They are more likely to get an infection and should be advised to receive a doctor's note, prior to you waxing them.

Obviously, if they are just getting a bikini wax or brow wax, then they can be waxed if they have varicose veins. But, a leg wax is not advised especially if they have a lot of them. If they only have a couple, just avoid the area and certainly don't wax over them.

Wax should not be applied over these areas:

- Raised moles and skin tags
- Any abrasions, bruises, bites, stitches, or broken skin
- Psoriasis, eczema (especially inflamed areas)
- Acne with infected pustules
- Any scars from surgery which are less than six months old (especially vasectomy scars as we *are* discussing waxing the berries!)

I once had a client who came in for a back wax. When I walked into the room and saw him lying face down waiting for me, I noticed his back was covered in long scratches on either side. I asked him if he had been wrestling a lion and what the heck had he done to his back! He informed me that he had a wild date the night before and she got a bit crazy during a night of passion!

I really wasn't comfortable applying wax onto his back as some areas were slightly inflamed. He insisted I waxed his back as he was going for round two that evening with the same girl and wanted to be 'groomed'! I really wasn't comfortable waxing him and told him so. I am sure he probably went to another salon down the street and got waxed. I lost the service and the client, but I was happier this way as it was a risk I wasn't willing to take.

Just like you would never give a client a facial with a cold sore, I would also never encourage you to do a lip wax on a client if she has one. It will certainly irritate the cold sore and is a sure guarantee that it will make it spread. It has been said to never wax a client if they are even susceptible to cold sores, regardless of whether they have an outbreak or not as it can trigger an outbreak. I am blessed once a year with the curse of cold sores and I receive waxes all the time and have never found this to be the case. From a holistic standpoint cold sores typically start from the base of the spine! Yes, they start from the nerve endings at the base of the spine; usually due to stress, being over tired which causes a low immune system or from too much sun without SPF lip protection. If you prefer in your salon to not offer waxing services to people who are *susceptible* to cold sores that is your call. Personally, if their outbreaks are once a year or once every couple of years, I would say it is pretty safe to go ahead with waxing. If they suffer from cold sores at least 5 times a year or more, it's probably best to not offer that service to them.

I also once had a client who came in for a back wax with a severe acne breakout. I consulted with him that applying wax would certainly irritate the skin, making his acne worse. I recommended that he received several back facials with me to help with the acne and then we could take it from there. I gained a new client and helped him with his acne which was a reward within itself. He soon became a waxing client once we had his acne under control. Knowing that he was a client with acne prone skin, we always used a cream wax specifically for sensitive skin.

Also, as mentioned earlier, if a client has a current genital herpes outbreak, then avoid waxing the genitals. Just out of courtesy, I would hope a client with a genital herpes outbreak, wouldn't *even* consider putting themselves or somebody else other than a doctor through that exposure anyway!

If a client is using Retin-A, Acutane, or any other medical grade topical cream for Acne, waxing is not recommended. This was discussed in detail in the prior section, The Questionnaire.

If your client is epileptic, has a pacemaker or metal implants just refrain from using high frequency following any waxing. I go into why this is crucial in the high frequency chapter.

Lip or brow waxing following a facial isn't necessarily a contraindication, but it's advisable to wax *before* a facial. The skin is super soft and beautifully hydrated and has more chance of lifting or being more sensitive due to the usage of steam, extractions, or exfoliation that it might have received.

If you do a lip or brow wax before a facial on your client, just avoid those freshly waxed areas with any harsh exfoliators.

I know this book is primarily about waxing the twigs and berries and our male clients are lucky to not have Aunt Flow visit once a month, so menstrual cycles are something that he doesn't need to worry about. I only mention this as it is not a contraindication to waxing but it does make us ladies more sensitive, both mentally and physically and it is worth you knowing this as some clients who are super hypersensitive choose to wait a few days before or after their period before receiving a wax. We can be crabby enough as it is during this time and really don't need the added pain thrown into the mix!

Nervous Client

If you have a nervous client, the best thing you can do is to talk to him. Ask him to describe his main concerns. Really listen to what he has to say, making eye contact with him to give him that reassurance that you are a caring aesthetician. If you show enough confidence, then he will very quickly confide in you. However, if a dithering aesthetician was fumbling around your bits, sweating profusely, and shaking her head in confusion due to total lack of confidence, wouldn't it make you want to grab your knickers and run right out of the room? I would!

As a professional technician, you must talk to your client confidently to help relieve any nerves that he may have. We are not checking out the goods and taking notes. We are just observing what we see so we can determine hair texture, skin, warts, moles or anything else that we see that we have to be prepared for ahead of time.

Your client is coming in to see you for an intimate close-up service so his bits and bobs will be exposed to you whilst you are performing the service. Some people like to cover the client up and work around a towel or disposable underwear to help keep their dignity somewhat in tact. Personally, I think all that fuss and stuff gets in the way of us trying to do our job. After all, your client has come in to have his pubic hair removed, so we need to do our job without stuff getting in the way of the nooks and crevices.

It's like going in for a haircut with a hat on and expecting your stylist to cut your hair around it because you are nervous about people seeing your bald patch. We are professionals and we are not there to stare at someone's anatomy and compare it to any other male client we saw previously that day. If he only wants the sides of his manhood waxed and not the whole nine yards, then, by all means, keep the disposable knickers on. Otherwise, don't bother with them because, again, if you are nervous about seeing his whole lunch box down there, then you are going to make him more nervous.

We should always show a certain amount of etiquette in the salon. If your client doesn't feel that he is getting that, then he, as a customer, is within his rights to express and voice his concerns and change salons or technicians. It is very important to really try to get the client to relax. The more relaxed he is, the more relaxed his muscles will be, which makes everybody happy and in the right frame of mind to do it again! So please, be confident in your approach. Be kind to the poor guy, and do your best as a professional to get him comfortable.

There are millions of Aesthetician out there, but it's the person, not the title as to why clients return.

Before the Procedure

Coffee, tea or any other stimulant all help us occasionally wake up in the morning or help us unwind after a long day, but consuming too much of any stimulant before a waxing appointment will only lead to more squirming, squealing, and discomfort. Why?

It's because our bodies become more acidic, and they certainly become more sensitive with an increase in blood flow, which, in turn, can make those berries turn more red than necessary. So, unless you want him to leave your room with his berries resembling two Rudolph's rubbing noses, please advise him prior to the appointment about his caffeine or alcohol consumption! Many a time, I have seen a client leaving a waxing service where he seriously looks as though he has not made it to the toilet in time because he is not walking properly. Thankfully, he wasn't gingerly walking out of my waxing room!

It is also a good idea to inform the client before his appointment that he can dull the nerve endings before the service by taking an aspirin or ibuprofen 20 minutes prior to his appointment. It really does help to do this, and I would highly recommend telling all of your clients this.

Also tell him to use a body scrub twice a week prior to waxing and to scrub around the pubic area to help 'exfoliate' those dead skin cells away from around the hair follicle. This helps ease the hairs exit, this also helps prevent ingrown hairs—especially if he continues to use it following the waxing procedure. If he doesn't have a body scrub at home, then this is a perfect time to show him your retail department and advise him on the best sugar scrub that he can buy.

Personally, I prefer that clients use a sugar scrub as opposed to a salt scrub (*unless they are using Epsom salts, which I cover in the "how to remove ingrown hairs section of the book*) Sugar is kinder on the skin and less dehydrating than salt. Also, rubbing salt into skin, especially around that area, is asking for trouble. Tell him to wait for 24 hours after his wax since rubbing sugar scrub into a freshly waxed area will be like rubbing your face up and down a hard bristle brush for five minutes. Exfoliating really does keep the follicle clean of dead skin, which then helps to discourage the hair from becoming ingrown.

I would advise against using a loofah due to their porous nature as they can harbour bacteria in the crevices. It is also surprisingly a good breeding ground for yeast to grow! They are also a bit too coarse for use in this area and should just generally be avoided.

It makes for a much better service if he hasn't shaved for at least two to three weeks so that the hair is long enough for the wax to grab onto. The hair ideally should be at least ¼ inches long. If the pubic hair is way too long and he looks like he is sporting a rain forest down there, then you might have to use clippers on it so it is easier to wax and less painful for him.

Some technicians do charge extra for using the clippers as it takes more time to complete the service. I prefer not to charge them as I feel it is all part of the preparation. You set the prices in your salon, so it is your call as to whether there is an add-on fee or not for clipping the hair down. But, I do think it is a good idea to have a variety of prices on our menu when waxing our clients. We don't charge per square foot, per se, but we should charge much more if he has never trimmed or waxed down there before. It will take you much longer to work through the jungle and this should be reflected in your pricing.

Another good reason for your client to not have super long hair down there is that when it is too long it might break at the surface of the skin (which is no different to shaving) and can break off during waxing. That hair needs to come out at the root.

Sometimes, when there are nice juicy roots with a big bulbous end, it can be pretty cool to show your client the waxing strip so that he can see that waxing is all worthwhile and, when done properly, it does work! Most clients don't like to see their own hair stuck to a muslin strip, but some do ask.

Ok, I know that skinny jeans have made a come back and, on some of our clients, they look great, but try and get him to leave those at home and opt for the loose, cotton trousers or sweat pants from his wardrobe instead. Chaffing isn't good after waxing and re-arranging the parts to avoid discomfort in the parking lot will scare away old ladies, which certainly isn't good, and will also encourage in-grown hairs, which is also not advisable.

So, advise your clients to arrive, clean and loose, and ready to breathe (physically and mentally). It is nice that they may want to smell all nice and sweet before they disrobe, but, hopefully, he will stay clear of the lotions and potions out of Grandma's medicine cabinet. Too much lotion can make it oily down under and we will prep the skin the professional way, not his way.

Consulting with your client about hair length, comfortable clothing and caffeine intake is always better when the receptionist makes the confirmation call or when initially booking the appointment. This isn't because the fashion police are prowling the salon or because we have more rules than we know what to do with. Instead, this is for the client's comfort, which should be our priority. It's just much better for him to know these simple instructions prior to coming into the salon, so he can plan ahead of time.

Claire Barnes

Act enthusiastic and you will be enthusiastic.
Dale Carnegie

Table Set-up

Here is what you need to have on-hand for your waxing service:

- Double wax heater or, if your room is large enough to hold a four-wax heater, all, the better . . . .
- Hard waxes
- Soft waxes
- Strips
- Hundreds of spatulas (as I don't recommend double dipping . . . nasty)
- Powder
- Prep oil
- Magnifying lamp
- Numbing spray (if you choose to use it prior to the waxing)
- Numbing lotion (if you choose to use it following the waxing)
- Disposable cleansing cloths
- Cleansing lotion
- Soothing lotion
- Latex gloves
- Sanitary wipes
- Tweezers (good aestheticians shouldn't rely on these . . . he's in for a wax, not a plucking!)

- Jar of Barbicide® (for sanitizing tweezers/clipper blades)
- Clippers (if he is sporting a 70's bush)
- Towels
- Cold wet towels (please see next page!)
- High frequency machine (if you want to spoil him!)
- Facial gauze (if using high frequency)

Tip 1: Cold Wet Towel

I put cold wet towels down for a reason, and I will go into that right now while it is fresh in your mind and before you get distracted.

Some men, whether they are gay, straight, attracted to you or not so attracted to you, can stand up to attention. And, by this, I mean that they can get an erection.
Now, before you get your knickers in a twist and run for the door, STOP and think that his 'winky' is re-known for being an involuntary muscle and has a mind of its own. There is some pulling going on down there, some attention is rustling around in his nether regions, and it just "does what it does" sometimes regardless of who is in its space.

Be professional about this, don't get flustered if this does happen, don't mention it or make a big deal out of it. If he's doing it for attention, he will love the extra attention and you are encouraging him to woo-woo his 'winky' for his sick pleasure, so the less attention you give him or IT, the better.

Kindly take your cold wet towel, place it over the area in question, tell him to think of his grandmother and turn your back and appear busy, cleaning up your cart and rearranging bottles like you do this all the time. Reassure him that this is common and it's no big deal. Make a big deal out of it and it will become a big deal. Most guys who come in for this service are not in it for sexual pleasure, but it can happen and you need to be prepared for it. In fact, I think I have only ever known this happen to me a handful of times. The men in question were not the most desirable characters and, luckily for me, I never saw them again.

To be blunt, they didn't get the "ending" they thought they were going to get so never returned again, which was fine with me. Going through some discomfort is usually pretty hard (excuse the pun) for a man to get an erection. In fact, it is the last thing on their mind and most men just want to get waxed and woo-woo their winkies all the way home again.

Remember, as a professional aesthetician, you are perfectly within your rights to end his service at any time if you feel that he is overstepping the boundaries. Perhaps, you could state this fact in print at the bottom of the questionnaire form.

You and your Salon can end a client's service at any time if you feel that they are drunk, stoned, or abusive towards you in any way that makes you feel uncomfortable.

So, now that we have the table set up, the room is of a comfortable temperature for both of you—not too hot, not too cold. This is for your comfort and also his, but it is also crucial to the temperature and application of the wax.

If he is too hot, he will sweat and trying to apply wax onto sweaty skin can make you sweat in frustration, which leads to a big sweaty situation and the room will resemble a skinned cat fight in a sauna.

If the room is too cold, he will be shivering, you will have ice cold hands even through the gloves, and the wax temperature can make the wax get too thick, which will be a blobby, stiff, and big sticky mess.

Out of courtesy to your client, I think it is always nice to check in with them about how comfortable they are in regards to the room temperature.

I also think it's nice to ask a client if they are happy with the music that you have playing. Most say "yes" and don't expect you to spin tunes like a top DJ and play requests for them, but it's nice for the client to be asked and it all makes for a top-notch customer service reputation for your salon or spa.

Admittedly, if it is not your own place of business but you are an employee with no choice as to what music is playing, then you are probably best keeping your mouth shut and not bringing attention to the situation so that you don't get into a pickle with your boss about his/her choice of music playing throughout the salon. But some employers allow you to have an iPod® docking station in your room where you can choose your own tunes, or better still if you rent the room, then, the music is all yours!

While we are on the subject of client comfort, please make it your duty to avoid phone calls during the service.

He may not be having a relaxing facial with dolphins playing in the background, but he is still spending money and expecting a service from you. Answering your cell phone or texting during any service is rude and is a sure guarantee that your client will not return.

If your phone accidentally bellows out the National Anthem, apologize to your client and switch your phone off or put it on silent! If you suspect it could be an emergency (as these do happen) then politely dismiss yourself to answer the call out of the room. If it isn't a life or death situation, return to the room promptly with the phone off and again apologize to your client.

I once felt like the third person during a hair cut that I had with a girl who took it upon herself to answer a personal phone call during my service. I was there for a service; I was short on time and felt that she was totally dismissive of my time while she chatted for a few minutes. It is not necessary and makes your client feel very unwanted. She began to proceed cutting my hair with "Ooh, where was I?" No apology, nothing! If you don't have a receptionist to make your appointments for you, allow your voicemail to take all messages and return them when you are in between clients.

Meeting Him at Reception/Salon Etiquette

Always greet your client with a nice smile and a relaxed confident, happy manner. If it is the first time that you are meeting him, you only have a few seconds to form a lasting impression so make sure you "wow" him with your pizzazz. The general public forms an opinion based on someone's looks within seven seconds. Even if it is your third time meeting the client, you should still treat him like he is your "only" client.

Become an actor in your environment and set the performance for each client that walks onto your stage. The most successful service technicians are ones that do this. They recognize that their personal problems have to be left at home and the stage has to be set and ready for action each time an existing or new client comes to you for a service.

The general public judges others based on looks, body language and attitude more than anything else. You have one chance to create a long lasting impression, so the rule as always is dress for success. Your appearance should be clean and very professional and your hair tied off your face if you have long hair. There should not be a trace of spinach in your teeth as, hopefully, you will have freshened up, and your smile should dazzle him to show him your true brilliance!

While we are on the subject of teeth, if you are a smoker it is strongly advisable to visit your dentist regularly. There is nothing worse than coming face to face with a person and their breath smells like they have had camel dung sandwich for lunch. So regardless of whether you smoke, or indulge in lots of garlic, keep a spare toothbrush at work with you to avoid any embarrassing halitosis moments!

An old beauty school teacher of mine once told us in class that most clients who visit salons or spas are spending at least $50 each visit, so, at the very least, you should look like you have spent at least that amount on yourself. Competition is very close to home. Winning your clients over within the first 20 seconds is crucial. We don't always get a second chance.

If your client enters the salon and you roll your eyes because the magazine that you were reading was at a juicy point and then you reluctantly throw your magazine down and, like a limp fish, shake his hand (if he is even lucky enough to get a handshake) and then mumble under your breath the introduction, you will have created an impression. The impression is "you are not that into your job, you don't care about him, and your magazine is way more interesting than what he is." Good job, sister!!

You must look at every client that walks through your door as your ideal client and treat them as such. Never make them feel that they are an interruption to your day or a big fat inconvenience. People who walk through your door are a word-of-mouth machine that can spread the word about your location, good or bad. At every point of engagement with your clients, you are essentially marketing your business.

You could do the best, most efficient service on him when he is in the waxing room, but his first impressions are what he encountered and are what he will remember. If your "meet and greet" skills are fantastic and your skill level is also fantastic in the waxing room, you are sure to get a repeat client and, better still, a client who recommends your services to his friends. Cha-ching!

So, be genuine and warm at all times. When you consider what each client means to your future and your bank account, then this shouldn't be so difficult. Practice these skills often enough and it will very soon become second nature. You will soon have it down to a fine art and you could do it whilst juggling hard boiled eggs and riding a unicycle in reception all at the same time and he won't even notice!! But, what he will notice are your fantastic etiquette skills and how you made him feel.

I learnt a very important lesson from somebody a while back who told me that "your brand is not your logo, it is not your company name, it is not necessarily what you wear (even though these all do contribute and play an important role), BUT it is how you made them feel!" This is who people buy from and this is what people remember when they think of you." Author Dale Carnegie once said "We are evaluated and classified by four contacts: what we do, how we look, what we say, and how we say it".

So, greet your client, shake his hand, and introduce yourself, making eye contact with him. Give him the reassurance he needs just by you being confident. Don't underestimate the power of using his name even if it is a difficult one to pronounce. Focus for a few seconds on the name or form a picture in your head to form an association with it so that you don't make the mistake of forgetting it. Some people understandably get upset if you keep forgetting their name.

During the service, use his name a couple of times to secure that you as a technician can bond with the client. Whenever I discuss etiquette in this book, I want you to always put yourself in your client's shoes and think of different scenarios that you may have encountered. Were you were made to feel neglected or unimportant? Or were you made to feel appreciated or overwhelmed by fantastic customer service? You decide which role you want to play in regards to how much salon etiquette you possess. Your client's safety and happiness followed by your retention rate, your bank account, and your tip jar is what should be important to you and all in that order.

It is reasonable to assume that if your tone of voice is happy, or excited, you will be able to project a more favourable impression than if your tone of voice is bored, frustrated, resentful or just tired. So, take the gum out of your pie hole, speak clearly and, hopefully with teeth free of spinach, you will have given him a good first impression. I could waffle on all day about spa/salon etiquette and how important it is today as I know what works and what doesn't.

I have worked in low-end salons to very high-end hotels and the rule applies everywhere. People do business with people they like and trust. Some of you reading this may be thinking, "What? Does she think I am an idiot? Of course I greet the client this way." But, surprisingly enough, not everybody does know or do this!! And, more importantly, some do it but not on a consistent basis. Some technicians (and I have had technicians who have done it to me) become complacent and become too familiar, treating me like I am their friend. You are not their friend as such; they are your client. At anytime, a client can decide, for whatever reason, that they want to go somewhere else. It could be due to financial issues, personal issues, or that they just merely want a change. Either way, it affects your back pocket and can become personal when it doesn't need to be. So, keep treating them at each visit, like it is their first visit.

I have been around the block often enough to come across the ones who "just don't get it!" So, my hopes are with writing this book, that those who just don't get it read this and think "maybe today is the day that I should get it, as the economy is tight, business might be going down the drain, and I need to step up to the plate and brush up on my people skills!"

Another big question you may have is "What do I address him by?" Do you call him "mister so and so?" Or do you address him by his first name. Your salon/spa will have its own branding and that should set the tone. Most high-end hotels require you to greet your clients in the spa by using "sir" or "mister so and so." Only you and your salon will know the correct way to address your clients.

Everyone has a brand and it is called your reputation. It really does determine how people respond to you and whether they will listen to you, buy from you and return back to you.

He trusts you, as a professional, to have an aura of confidence about you. Shaking hands whenever conducting business dictates you are forming a relationship with him. The service should end this way when he is at the reception area also so that you give the impression that you are grateful for his business with the hopes of seeing him again. Incidentally, take note that after having his berries waxed his hands may be slightly clammy due to nerves (don't grimace at him as your hands were touching his nether regions earlier; the poor guy needs a break!).

If you appear all flustered before you even begin or are traumatized before the whole event, he will pick up on this and flee the salon, burning rubber as he accelerates out of the parking lot. Also, another point I would like to make is that when greeting him in reception, unless your reception area looks like a morgue and there are no other clients there, please, please don't shout out loud, "So you are here today to see me for a "back, sack, and crack wax?"

You know the feeling when you go into the doctor's office and the receptionist who might be as dumb as a box of frogs yells over the counter, "So you are here to see the Doctor for what exactly?" You mumble in a whisper that you are here to see him for the irritable bowel issue as all the rubber-neckers in the waiting area strain to hear your medical history.

So, the point that I am trying to make is he doesn't want to hear the sniggers from the other guys or girls in there who might be waiting for a pedicure or just a hair trim. Keep it respectful, respect his privacy, and think how you would feel. The ins and outs of his service can be discussed once he is in the room, and I will go into that a bit later as this does need to be discussed just to make sure he's at the right place for the right service.

*We are given two ears and one mouth for a reason . . . .
use what we are given wisely. Epictetus*

Client Hygiene

Okay, we don't care how great a footballer our client is or how big his shlonker is or how handsome he might be, but could you please make sure that he gets it clean before he disrobes and exposes his manly tackle, lunch box, or whatever term you like to call it.

We love our clients and appreciate their business and we also care about their well-being as we remove hair from the wobbly, sensitive bits, but we DON'T wish to see deposits left from his last make-out session or last bathroom visit. Believe me, in our careers, we have or we will see this, so to avoid any embarrassment on our part, please get him to wipe up properly with the baby wipes that you provide for him so that he can refresh his nether regions and let us begin.

When leaving the room, to give him a bit of privacy, you should provide him with a towel to cover up with, so that the crown jewels are not exposed to the whole salon or to anybody just casually walking past the door! Our gynaecologist sees us naked from the waist down, but they don't stay in the room and watch us undress. They leave the room and provide a cover up to protect us from a lost patient accidentally walking into the room or passers by peeking in. So, to protect your client's nudity against strays walking in accidentally, leave the towel so he can cover up.

Point him towards the box of baby wipes before you leave the room, so that he can wipe down with them and dispose of it in the labelled trash can next to the massage bed. The baby wipes and tissues are provided for this reason only and under no circumstances should you, as a professional, allow him to abuse your intellect by his hinting, suggesting, or presuming that a happy ending will take place. If this is what you think he is looking for, I am sure you can point him in the right direction to a more appropriate place of his choice. Keep our industry clean. Earn your tips the correct way.

Client Consultation

Make sure the guy is in there for a Brazilian wax and not just a chest wax! We all know from time to time that our very busy wonderful receptionists can make a mistake or things are just misunderstood over the phone. The last thing you need is to start prepping his downstairs department when he is wondering what the heck this has to do with a chest or back wax! He doesn't want any surprises!

Consult with him as to what his requirements are whilst he is in the room. Does he need a full back, sack and crack wax or does he just want a modest clean up around the sides and top? Maybe he wants a trendy landing strip left and the berries are left in tact? Listen to what his requirements are and advise whenever possible if you have any other recommendations.

Most guys who come in for this service require the whole nine yards and want you to wax everything in his nether regions. But, it is your job to find out this information and not to assume. Whenever we ASSUME . . . You basically make an ASS out of U and ME!).

I will share a story with you that happened to me years ago when the Brazilian first became popular with females. I met my client in the reception area and she was booked in for a Brazilian wax. She was a rookie to the service and obviously when booking her appointment thought that the Brazilian was just a simple bikini wax.

During the procedure, I started to ferret my way through her lady garden, removing every inch of her pubic hair, whilst she was positioned in every yoga position known to man. She then started to panic and got slightly upset as she sat upright and, with a total look of sheer horror on her face, told me that she only wanted the sides done around her bikini area and then asked me why I insisted that she roll over so I could get her back passage!

I stood, rooted to the spot with the deer in headlights look on my face and with mouth gaping wide open like I was catching flies! I kept glancing down at the trash can, overflowing with spatulas and used wax strips with the hopes that somehow, just somehow, I could miraculously glue it all back on again and make it all right.

With my bottom lip quivering, I attempted to start explaining what I thought she was in for and that she should have been more clear during her time of booking the appointment, BUT I stopped myself before I made her feel like I was the victim. So, I just outright humbly apologized and told her how bad I felt that I didn't take the time to double check with her what exactly she was in for.

Some people have a hard time apologizing and are very quick to point the blame at others. We cannot do this with our clients, we have to treat them like they are right . . . as difficult as it can be, it is detrimental to your business if you blame your clients and make them feel that they are in the wrong.

My consultation in the room didn't even take place, and I failed miserably! There was obviously no charge to the client. I didn't see her again and neither did I get a tip. Actually, yes, I did get a tip. The tip is CONSULT with your client what their needs are! Be clear before you start, so he isn't left resembling a plucked turkey for Thanksgiving as maybe he just wants to leave feeling like he still looks like an adult and not a new born baby.

Client Responsibility

Even though he may be paying top dollar for the service and may think he just has to lay there and think of England/America or whatever country he is from, he has to work with you so that he gets the best, quickest, and less painful encounter ever. By this I mean he is responsible for holding, stretching, and pulling the twig, the scrotum, his bum cheeks apart and everything else that needs rearranging down there. This is to help keep the skin as taut as possible.

The more confident you are when using certain terminology, the better. If you use words that make you sound like you are embarrassed, shy, and nervous about what you are doing, he will tense up like a possum, play dead, and it will be like working on a corpse. And, for goodness sake, don't talk to him in a sing-song voice with cutesy little nicknames for his twig. He will feel like his grandmother is rustling around his junk, cooing to him like he is a baby.

One of the other reasons why I suggest that he is responsible for holding his twig and stretching it from one end of the room to the other as you work around the area is there is less chance he has of standing to attention. If you get that golden tool in your hand, start rubbing it, soothing it, and just generally playing with it like it is play dough, the more it is likely to get erect, time slows down, the cold towel has to come out and it makes your job so much harder (excuse the pun).

Be firm (again, excuse the pun!) but be nice with him. But, more importantly and I cannot say this enough, be confident and make him feel special. As in all walks of life, the more confident we are as individuals, the more confidence we instil in others and the more we make people feel special the more likely they are to return to us.

The customer in every walk of business has to be made to feel like he is your only customer. If you accomplish this, you will be very successful. Even if your client has been a client for years, he should still be made to feel this way.

Complacency breeds ignorance, which affects our bottom line.

If he has never had any "manscaping" before down there and his bush resembles something out of a 1970's movie, it is strongly suggested that you get the clippers out or hedge trimmer, weed-wacker, or whatever you can get your paws on. Trim it down to a No. 2. As I mentioned earlier, if the hair is too long, it can break off at the skin's surface, so a nice ¼ inch is the ideal hair length. If your client has super coarse hair as some different ethnic groups do, then a nice ½ inch length is probably better.

So, once the consultation is out of the way and the possible trimming and he knows the protocol, then it's time to get down to the nitty-gritty and begin prepping the skin for the application of wax.

Why We Wear Gloves

As we enter the room and our client is lying there with the towel over him, clean and wiped down from the baby wipes—we then put on our latex gloves. We do not remove the towel, take a peek, and then put on the gloves. I strongly suggest putting your gloves on 'before' you remove the towel that is guarding the jewels. Why before?

Think about this—if somebody was to remove the towel from your bits, take a peek, and then put on the latex, you would be thinking "hmmm, do I look like I have something going on down there that needs the latex?" So, before you engage in physical contact with your client, out of professionalism, please do this. You will actually be surprised as to how many technicians don't wear gloves during waxing as they find they get in the way, get sticky, and just annoy the heck out of them.

Again, think of the gynaecologist. They should have their gloves on before they remove our paper sheet, and they certainly don't go touching our downstairs Lady Garden without gloves on. Neither should you! Latex gloves protect us from diseases, blood spots, and Hepatitis C.

Latex gloves also protect the client. The nails, no matter how short they are, are a wonderful source of bacteria. The most common bacteria found under the nail bed are 'staphylococcus.' It is nasty and can cause various skin diseases, including 'impetigo,' which is extremely contagious and spreads very quickly. Impetigo occurs when there is a break in the skin, but can also occur if there is no visible break in the skin. Bacteria enter and grow there, causing inflammation and infection. Blisters occur and fill with pus; it is very unsightly and can be pretty painful.

When the hair is pulled from the root, it is very susceptible to infection. Wearing the latex gloves helps eliminate as much of this as possible. Blood spots can also occur with any type of waxing, which is a good, enough reason in itself to wear gloves. If you do find your gloves get a bit sticky whilst waxing, sprinkle a bit of baby/corn powder over them, rub your hands together, and it will help with the tacky feeling. Hopefully, you won't be on such a tight budget that a fresh pair can't be replaced also.

Even though we are wearing gloves when we wax, it is also a good idea to double check that our immunizations are up to date. As aestheticians work so closely with the skin and sometimes use sharp implements like lancets* during facials (*depending on the State you are licensed in) it's advisable to have a Tetanus Shot, and a Hepatitis A and B shot. Unfortunately there is no shot available at the time of writing this book for Hepatitis C.

Hepatitis is a virus that is found in infected blood, semen, vaginal fluids and saliva. The disease causes liver damage, long term disease, liver cancer and death.

If an aesthetician waxed me wearing gloves, I would also consider going to see her for facials, if she did indeed offer this service. If she didn't wear gloves and tried to introduce me to a new facial service she was offering with a wonderful discount, I would most certainly refrain from taking her up on her offer. Who knows how many Lady Gardens, or Twigs and Berries she had touched that day!? As aestheticians we all know to wash hands before and after every new client, but I don't want to take the risk, in case it just 'slipped' her mind!

People soon forget how fast you did a job, but they remember how well you did it forever.
Howard W Newton

Skin Prepping

Make sure your facial/massage bed is at a comfortable height for you to begin waxing. Ergonomics are something we should always take into account. If your bed is too low and you find that you are bending down constantly, it can affect your health over the long term. Ideally, flat shoes should be worn and not heels (I can be guilty of this occasionally as I just love heels), but, ideally, flat shoes are better for the posture when waxing all day.

The lighting in the room should be sufficient enough also, so that it doesn't strain your eyes and the better the lighting the more hairs that you can see. Use your magnifying light during the waxing and also during the skin prepping time to check the area for hair growth patterns, or anything that might look dodgy!

Use a nice skin prep solution. I recommend one from Cirepil® called Cristal, which is really nice and it cleans the skin maintaining the skins acid mantle without stripping it of its good natural oils. Using your cleansing cloth and prep solution, clean the area thoroughly to make sure the surface is clean and free from bacteria and also free from oil that the body naturally produces from its sebaceous glands.

Don't use a toner or astringent (certainly not alcohol!!) as this will tighten up those little pores and squeeze the living daylights out of the hair follicle, which will make it harder to pull out the hair from its follicle. It also makes the skin too dry, which can cause lifting (another word for saying 'pulling off the skin').

A nice warm towel over the area can be applied prior to the skin prep solution. This can help relax the client, but the warmth can actually help soften the pores, which helps ease the hair out of the follicle. So, killing two birds with one stone can only make your life and his life easier.

There are two ways to prep the skin prior to waxing: Prep oil or baby powder/corn starch. Some clients also like you to use a numbing spray before you start waxing them. Gigi® has a great topical analgesic spray that gently desensitizes the skin as it has 4% Lidocaine in it, which minimizes the discomfort within minutes. Gigi® also has one for sensitive skin if your client is of the sensitive nature! If it is their first time—and I can tell that they are nervous—then I always use it before I wax. I tell the client that I am using it so that it helps to relieve some of the sting for them.

They do appreciate this extra kindness that you put into the service, and all the little extra things that you do will make him more likely to return to you and become more generous in the tipping department.

Of course, you are always going to come across a client who is as tight as a drum no matter what you do and moths fly out of their wallets when money has to be spent. Don't take it personally; as it is not always down to you, it is just the way that they are.

Oil

Ok, now some people like to use prep oil before waxing. Some of you may be asking, "prep oil before waxing? How can oil be applied to the skin before waxing?"

The reason we apply oil before waxing is to ensure that the skin is protected and only the hair is removed. After all, removing skin isn't what he is in for. If he was, he would be down at the plastic surgeon and having a skin lift or graft. We are here to wax and not remove the skin. Cirepil® has lovely prep oil, which has a nice aroma to it and is fantastic at prepping the skin. Use it very, very sparingly.

Also, some aestheticians like to use just powder before waxing and both are okay as it is all just a matter of preference.

Personally, I find that every client is different. I can usually tell this by their ethnic background. If they have what seems like oily skin, then I will apply powder as oily skin and prep oil is just a bad combination. Again, it is all just a case of what you are comfortable with.

You will probably find that you steer towards one more than the other. I certainly prefer to powder up the scrotum more than using oil. I do explain later why I prefer powder on the scrotum. Another benefit of powder that I find is that it shows up the hairs making them more visible, which makes for a more thorough service.

When applying oil to the skin prior to waxing, use a tiny amount. Put it in the palm of your hands, blot your hands against a clean towel to prevent too much application, and start dabbing the area down there with your palms to be waxed. If it feels too slick and shiny after you have applied it and he is starting to look like a professional wrestler from Turkey (that is a national sport in Turkey by the way, where they rub themselves in olive oil and wrestle their opponent!), then you have probably applied too much. So, using a towel again, dab around the area to absorb any excess oil. The skin shouldn't feel oily at all. Neither should you see it glisten. In this case, less is better.

Powder/corn starch

Powder adheres to the hair and protects the skin. This is a perfect prepping method to use on areas that need to be waxed where the skin is thin or sensitive. Powder is used on eyebrows, lips, and bikini areas to protect the skin from lifting.

When applying powder to the skin prior to waxing, use a light mist over the area so that you just coat the area lightly. If you use too much powder, the wax will form a sort of curdle-like consistency and it will just result in a poor application with bad hair removal. You can sprinkle the powder from the container over large body parts when waxing, but when waxing the facial area, always, always, apply powder to eyebrows or lips from powder sitting in your hand, never directly from the container itself!

Tell your client what you are doing and why just out of courtesy and also as a confidence booster. He will appreciate you telling him the reasons why you are applying powder and why you are doing what you are doing. Clients don't make a point of doing business with technicians that they dislike, don't trust, or whom they have no respect for.

Applying the Wax

There are lots of different waxes to use. Soft wax comes in lots of different types, depending on hair textures/skin sensitivity, etc. If you are lucky enough to have a wax heater that holds several different pots of wax, then you can really play around with the different types of wax and enjoy seeing how they all work in relation to each client with different hair textures, etc.

One of my favourite soft waxes that I love is one from Cirepil® called Blanche. I love the smell and the consistency and, to be honest, could see it spread on toast as it resembles pale golden honey. But, I will refrain from licking it as I am sure it looks way better than it would taste.

Briefly discuss with your client the sort of wax you are using and why. Keep it to layman's terms and don't bore him with the chemistry of the wax (even if you know it). He just wants the simple facts without the fuss. Explaining to him which wax you are going to use and why will tell him that you are quite capable of doing your job and have it all under control. It also shows that you care about him and his well-being.

So, you have prepped his skin and his jewels are ready to be worked on, so now you can start your job.

When applying soft wax on a male client around his privates, I always work around the twig with him holding it at all times like I mentioned earlier. He is responsible for pulling it, adjusting it, and allowing me to work around it. Tell him to hold it like it's a joy stick and he is playing Xbox®, moving it around to make your job quicker and much less embarrassing for him. He can pull it really hard to allow you to apply wax and remove the wax whilst the skin is being kept taut.

Two reasons I do this is: So that he knows how far to pull without hurting himself *and* it keeps the skin taut to make removal much easier. However, the most important thing is the more you grab hold of it and pull it around like it's your own joy stick, the inevitable is going to happen and the cold towel will have to come out!

Be professional and save him some embarrassment and the least amount of discomfort as you can. This method also applies to the clean-up process when you are applying lotion to remove some excess wax or to just soothe the skin. During this time, it is especially important that he is in control of keeping the joy stick firmly under grips!

So, instruct him in a friendly manner what his role is in the service so that you can then begin to apply the application of the wax and begin his service.

Now, remember to use a clean spatula each time you dunk into the wax pot as double dipping can cause contamination. I say 'can' because I don't think it has ever been proven that double dipping has done this before.

To be on the safe side, I would stick with (excuse the pun) the State Board rules and regulations and get into the habit of using clean spatulas/sticks for each dip just to prevent cross contamination if nothing else. *I do go into detail a bit later in the book about the importance of no double dipping.* I wouldn't like to think I was having an eyebrow wax with wax that had earlier been in contact with some guy's scrotum or a not so clean lady garden!

I personally like to start from the top and work my way down, using soft wax around the pubic area leaving a few inches in a circular shape around the twig where I later apply the hard wax. When applying soft or hard wax around this area, his twig should be pulled taut from side to side or pulled downwards. This area and the bum cheeks are the only part of the Brazilian wax where I use soft wax (with strips).

Always test the temperature of the wax on your inside wrist before you begin. It should be as close to body temperature as possible. If it feels hot to the touch, then it is too hot to apply to the downstairs body parts or any part of the body for that matter. Turn the temperature down if it is too hot and leave it to cool slightly with the lid off. If the wax also literally drips off the spatula and is of a very runny consistency, that is a good guideline that the wax is too hot to apply to the body also.

The same rule applies to hard wax also. Hard wax at the right temperature is easy to roll around the spatula, leaving a bulbous blob at the end with no rapid dripping. If the hard wax in the tin is the same consistency and all runny, it is also too hot. Hard wax at the right temperature has a thicker centre with the outside less firm, but certainly not drippy!

When you have the soft wax at the perfect temperature, you can then begin waxing your client. Dip your clean disposable spatula into the wax. On the one side of the stick, wipe the excess off on the side of the waxing rim. Hopefully, you have a paper collar around the pot to catch any drips. A soiled, sticky pot is also a good breeding ground for bacteria and a State Board faux pas, so use a paper collar and change it frequently.

Apply a thin layer of soft wax to the skin, holding the stick at a 45 or a 90-degree angle, and with the other hand, stretch the skin ever so lightly as you do this so that the spatula doesn't drag and blob too much wax in one place onto the skin. As you hold the skin taut, the wax application is thinner and this makes hair removal so much better. Whilst you are applying the wax, your client is holding himself and pulling his twig to keep it out of the way and to help with keeping the skin around the area that you are waxing taut. Holding the skin taut whilst applying wax and removing wax helps to prevent hickies, love bites, or what ever term you are familiar with.

Hold the skin around the area that you are about to wax and pull taut whilst applying the wax in the direction of the hair growth. Apply wax in very small sections until you pick up your speed. If you apply wax to the hair in the opposite direction to the natural hair growth pattern, as you pull the strip off, it will break the hair at the surface, leaving dark spots (these are not blackheads, but broken hair).

Keep your sections small and continue checking on the direction of the hair growth when applying the wax. Personally, I much prefer to use muslin (fabric) strips when working on the bikini area. I find it folds into the genital area much easier and seems gentler on the skin. Some people prefer to use paper strips and, again, that is fine as it's all down to personal preference.

When waxing the bikini area on a male or female, there is no need to use long waxing strips. Keep your strips around 5" long. If your strip is around 12" long, like it would be if you were doing a leg or back wax you will have lots of waste and not have as much control as you would do if it was shorter. When the strip is shorter you are able to remove the strip with perfect parallel control. When it is this short you will still be able to have at least 1/3 of the strip free to use as your clean fold, to hold onto when removing the strip.

Glide your hand over the strip towards the hair growth, avoiding rubbing up and down with your hand like you are expecting a genie to appear. Going back and forth is unnecessary and can cause the hair under the strip to weaken and break off. Ever removed a strip before and seen broken hair at the surface? This occurs because of one or two things: Either you rubbed the strip too much, causing the hair to weaken and break off, or when you pulled the strip off, you lifted it away from the body, flicking it practically across the room and are left to peel it off the ceiling or the wall opposite to you.

Incidentally, the only time that I do rub the strip like I am expecting a genie to appear, is when I wax the top of my clients feet, during a leg wax. A lot of the time the strip is removed and the wax sticks to the feet because they are cold. I rub the strip to warm the feet up a bit to make it easier to remove. If this still doesn't work, I tuck my fingers under the edge of wax and remove the strip and wax that way, to help ease it from the feet instead. Or I get them to wear socks until I am ready to wax that area to keep them warm.

So, once you have applied the strip and glided your hand across it towards the direction of the hair growth, remove the strip as 'parallel' (close) to the skin as possible. As you do this, your wrist should cause a flicking motion or a punching out of the hand. When waxing any part of the body using soft wax, you always keep the strip as close as possible to the skin when removing it. Do this and watch those fat bulbous roots appear on the strip which is what you want. Show your client, frame the darn thing, pat yourself on the back and know that those suckers have come out from their hiding place. When the strip and hair from the patch you have just worked on has been removed, apply firm pressure to the area to relieve some of the 'sting'.

You don't need to use a new strip each time, but once the strip has become quite thick with wax, dispose of it and use a new one. Too much wax sitting on the wax strip might save you some money as you won't be going through lots of them, but it doesn't always grip the hair as well as it should do if it is caked with wax residue.

Talk with your client. Try to get to know him by asking questions about his family, hobbies, etc. It keeps their mind distracted, and most men love to talk about themselves! It builds trust also if you show an interest. Ask him what he does for a living and if he lives locally. If you don't get much of a response and he seems reluctant to talk, pay attention to this. He may be shy or he may not want to answer your questions, so don't take it personally.

If he is unresponsive, then quit the chatting, read his body language and just work in silence if that is what you think he needs. Don't take this as a cue for you to start talking about your life or your latest boyfriend/girlfriend break up. There is nothing worse than a technician who keeps on waffling non-stop about herself and her life . . . drama, drama, drama. Keep it for those who may want to listen outside of work, but don't bring it into your client's space.

Our clients have personal lives and we don't always know what is happening in their life. They may come to your salon as an escape and a getaway from their hectic, stressed life. Make their experience a pleasant one without them feeling the burden of having to listen to you! This doesn't just apply in the waxing room, but should be a genuine rule of thumb in the service industry, period.

He may not want to make small talk or listen to small talk, but you still need to speak to him as you are informing him each time with what direction you need him to pull his twig. He doesn't understand the waxing pattern or your pattern of waxing; he needs to know what his job is during the process.

Even if your client isn't in the large shoe department club, he still needs to hold his twig and pull it around to keep it from flopping in your work area.

Oh, and incidentally, please don't tell him that he isn't in the club!

I once had a client whose twig was inverted. This is not very common and you may never come across it. I believe it is a condition that can be caused by circumcision and usually rectifies itself over time. With my client, this obviously wasn't the case. He was also heavy set, and I have learnt that too much fat around the area can cause it to have an inverted appearance causing him to lose an inch or two. If he doesn't have a twig per se to pull and stretch, he will still need to stretch the surrounding skin around this area, just like he does with his scrotum, to allow the skin to be kept taut.

We just do our job as normal without making any reference to our client's misfortunes or disabilities as we are professionals and non judgemental to his physique.

Tip 2: Cold Wet Towel Again!

Another tip that I do that I would like to share with you in regards to the really sensitive clients is to apply pressure after each pull with a cold damp wash cloth over the area to help take the sting out. This is a pretty good tactic for the first time client and, yes, this can be time-consuming and more work for you, but if you do this and they appreciate the extra kindness and care you put into their service, they are more likely to come back to you. My clients particularly of Middle Eastern descent like to receive this during a back or chest wax as their hair tends to be much thicker and coarser.

Most men (sorry guys, but it's pretty true) can be big babies and they do love the extra care that we put into caring for them. Use this to your advantage and watch the client retention rate increase and your tip jar overflow. Inform your client that you are doing this for him to help him out a bit and that you are giving him some 'extra' care. In return, you will be far more memorable in his eyes than a technician who speed waxes him like she has a rocket up her bum and just wants his money so that she can move onto the next victim.

Too many technicians speed wax and boast about the speed that they complete the service in, overlooking whether care has gone into the service or whether all the hair has been removed. Plenty of clients have told me that some techs made them feel rushed, that hair was still left in the grooves, and that driving home, their right testicle felt like a Brillo pad. Consequently, they didn't go back and that aesthetician has lost a potential repeat client all because speed and money were more important than doing a good job. What comes around goes around as the saying goes.

A Bit about Hair Growth Stages

Without boring you about the anatomy of the hair cycles, I will keep this brief. It is worth you knowing the basics, so you and your client can understand why they may get re-growth in a couple of days after their wax. Hair, that starts to grow back immediately following a wax is not hair that was waxed today, but hair that was just underneath the surface of the skin that you couldn't necessarily see.

It always confused me in beauty school when I was given too many scientific terms associated with hair and it's growth stages, hence the reason I am keeping it simple and trying to get the message across in simple to understand terminology without you falling asleep and drooling at the mouth from boredom.

In an ideal world of waxing and what I picked up in beauty school was that clients should begin their appointments: On day one, then on day 15 and then again on day 30 for five months. They then start their waxing appointments around the fifth month on a monthly basis. As they approach the seventh month, repeat the one day, fifteenth day, and the thirtieth day process again for one month, and then back to monthly appointments.

Confused? As I said, this is in an ideal world and we all know how difficult it can be at times to get our clients to commit to such a schedule and can also be costly for them. But, if you can get them to follow this routine, then it is even better for their hair growth patterns and will produce better results.

Try it on yourself at home and see if you like it, it makes it easier to 'sell' this idea to your clients and helps you articulate it better to them when you educate them on their own hair growth patterns. Practice what you preach and experience this method yourself to understand the difference it makes when doing it this way.

Hair has three growth cycles:

Anagen (hair bulbs are found nestled in the subcutaneous fat)
Catagen (hair bulbs are found in the dermis)
Telogen (hair bulbs are found in the upper dermis)

During the three stages of hair growth, the bulb is found in different positions as you can see above.

Anagen: This is the active/growing phase and can last for at least three weeks. The cells are dividing rapidly as they sit in the subcutaneous fat, way down deep where we cannot see it. The amount of time it stays in this phase is generally genetically determined. Approximately 85% of all hairs are in the growing phase at this time.

Catagen: This hair is getting ready to shed as it is approaching the dermis and is coming towards the end of the hair growth. It is during this stage that the hair shrinks. Maybe it doesn't want to see daylight and starts to whither away? A bit like me on a Monday morning I suppose!

Telogen: The hair is now resting and is a dead, fully keratinized hair. This is the hair that we see and quite obviously doesn't like daylight as it dies before it get's to this stage! At the end of this phase if the old hair has not already been shed, the new hair pushes it out and the hair growth cycle starts all over again.

Tip 3: What to Do If the Hair Is A Bit Short

Ideally a client should wait at least two to three weeks since shaving, or his last wax before his next appointment as the hair is usually not long enough for the wax to grab hold of. But sometimes, a client may come in and his hair is slightly too short in just some places and you don't think the wax will remove all of it. To understand this a little bit more refer back to the previous chapter on hair growth stages.

What I was trained to do during my 2,000 hours of training in the U.K. by my wonderful teacher, was to apply the wax against the hair growth. Then, using the same spatula so as not to apply it too thickly, immediately apply the wax towards the hair growth. Apply the muslin strip as normal, glide the hand towards the hair growth and remove the strip parallel to the skin as usual. In this way, the motion with the wax on the stick is back and forth.

No double dipping has occurred; it simply means that wax has been applied in two different directions to coat both sides of the hair. The final application of wax is applied towards the hair growth so the hair doesn't just break off at the surface of the skin upon removal which is pointless during waxing. It is also one of the main reasons why ingrown hairs occur.

Remember, no genie rubbing against the strip; a firm glide is sufficient! This method of waxing against the hair growth is only used when the hairs are teeny tiny and the goal is to remove them without relying on tweezers.

Pre-warn the client that the tiny hairs might be an issue to remove but that you have a technique up your sleeve to help shift the buggers out of their hiding place. Again, sharing this with him will make you more memorable in his eyes, and he will have the confidence that you can rectify problems, come up with a Plan B, and that you put the extra time into his care. This shows professionalism.

Even though the hairs might have been double-sided with wax and you removed the strip correctly, they still might not want to budge. This is when the tweezers have to come out (which I hate). Most clients would prefer to have their bottom impaled by a cactus rather then experience having their nether regions tweezed!

Any technician who spends more time with the tweezers in her hand than the wax needs to re-train or find a job on a farm, plucking chickens. So, if you think that you are one of those secret hair tweezers, keep reading this book, get some more training, or ask for help from your work colleagues. Any successful person is always willing to help others out also. We become successful by helping others to be successful too. It's just plain good karma!!

Tip 4: Hair Growth Patterns Down Under

A general rule of thumb, which is not set in stone but is usually pretty accurate, is what I like to refer to as the North, East, South, West factor. Take a look at your own Lady Garden and look at the hair growth. From the pubic bone area, the hair tends to be heading south even though it is in the north sector of the nether regions. Underneath your Lady Garden up the lip/labia, it tends to grow inwards east or west, depending on whether we are looking at the right lip or the left lip.

From the bum hole and some of the labia, it is in the south sector but is growing up to the north. As I said, this isn't set in stone, but, as a guideline, keep it in mind so you get your speed and pattern down a bit better and observe the hair growth as you go.

On a man, the hairs around his twig grow downwards and towards the centre of his stomach, and the hairs around his scrotum tend to grow upwards. Again, this isn't set in stone, but you do start to see that it's pretty much a pattern amongst our clients.

So, working from the top of the pubic area, I like to work in sections. The side that I am working on around his pubic area and thigh area, I have him angle his leg in a V position so that his heel is parallel to his knee across from his straightened leg. This makes the skin tighter whilst working around it and applying wax. I work around the area, moving towards his thigh and bikini line section.

If he is a pretty toned client with good muscle structure, I can pull the skin taut myself when applying wax and removing it. With the larger built client, who may have more folds or just looser skin around his body, I always get him to hold the skin taut and pull it tightly. I guide his hands as to where I want them and kindly tell him what I would like him to do for me and why. This just simply makes your job easier and it makes it less painful for him, which is more important than how easy it is for you and it also avoids bruising.

I then come down towards the thigh area and, wanting to remove some hairs around this area going towards his genitals, I come across the beast called the 'tendon'! I am sure some of you, during your training at beauty school, caused a bruise whilst waxing and was left wondering what the heck you did wrong! Or, you had a bikini wax once and you came out with what resembled a hickey or a love bite on your inner thigh! Try explaining that one to your partner! The tendon is the sensitive structure on the inside of the thigh, which is extremely sensitive and bruises very easily. I will go into how to wax around the tendon in the next chapter.

Once you have finished working from the top of the bikini and around the side, thigh and tendon area, repeat the process on the other side of the shaft. Get your client to hold his leg in the V position again on the side that you are working on and keep getting him to hold the thigh area or his belly area taut to help you in the process.

Once the area around the twig is hair free, there should be a little patch of hair around the twig about an inch in diameter that you have left. I remove this hair with hard wax (stripless wax) as the very base of the twig is very sensitive for most clients as the hair is denser. Dust more powder over this area if there is no traces of powder there and with the client pulling his twig in a downward stretch, (possibly tucking it underneath if he is in the large shoe department club) apply the hard wax and remove the wax against the direction of the hair growth. Pulling himself downwards gives you a good taut stretch of the skin and gives you plenty of room to manoeuvre your hands when removing the wax.

Think of your own pubic bone if you are a female reading this and you have had a full Brazilian wax before. This area is super sensitive for most people. It hurts way more than having the labia lovely Lady Garden done, so be conscious of this area and be sensitive to his needs. He doesn't have a pubic bone like we do, but it still hurts, due to the hairs density.

Some clients have hair actually growing down their twig also. DO NOT use soft wax on this area. Always powder it up well and apply hard wax with the help of the client who holds himself. This makes the application and removal so much better for the client and for you as the technician.

Tip 5: Bruises/Hickey Prevention

It's important to pay special attention to the tendon area at all times when waxing and to keep the client's leg in its comfortable V section. The wax is applied down the thigh as the hair in this area tends to grow downward (Think N, E, S, and W!). Apply the wax thinly over that area, keeping the skin taut as you would do normally. Then, apply the strip to the area and, with your other free hand that is keeping the skin taut prior to removing the strip you, tuck a couple of fingers UNDER the tendon.

Pull the strip parallel to the skin, keeping the skin firm but gently with your fingers pressed UNDER the tendon while releasing the strip. Do this properly each time and no bruising will take place. Keep practicing and feeling around under your own tendon, find that little groove section where you can press into it. This area tends not to hurt when pressed underneath, but it does bruise easily if left exposed with no grip protection when a strip of wax is being pulled from it. Always keep the wax application as thin as possible also. If it is too thick, it takes extra work on the skin to remove it, which can also aid in bruising. When using this method, the same applies if you were using hard wax in this area too.

Bruising looks unsightly and shouldn't happen. If it does happen (as accidents can and do happen), explain and apologize to the client immediately that this has occurred. Most of the time, they are okay with it. They may not be over the moon and doing cartwheels naked around your room in excitement because they are leaving with a hickey, but, if you are polite enough and have acknowledged it whilst sweetly saying 'sorry,' then you may be forgiven. If you send them out of the door without so much as an apology, they will be left thinking this is a normal part of the service and, chances are, you won't be seeing them again.

I have another story to share with you. During a female Brazilian waxing service, I didn't pay enough attention to this area. Chatting away to my client like I had verbal diarrhoea, I overlooked the necessity to pay extra attention around that area. I was fresh out of beauty school and wanted to cry when I discovered what happened. I got all hot and flustered. I wanted to flee from the room, grab my stuff, and get the heck out of there never to be seen again apart from on the back of a milk carton or under the missing person's section!

My mouth became as dry as a bone and I seriously froze on the spot as that bruise appeared instantly on the surface of the skin like an illuminated light bulb, blinking at me. I was left rooted to the floor, hoping just by some miracle it would disappear or that I would just disappear. I very humbly said, "I am so sorry, but I think when I removed the strip of wax, my pressure must not have been as firm as it should have been and it has caused a bruise around your bikini line."

I wasn't met with a smack in the face, but just greeted by a little face from my client, peering between the legs into the bikini area to examine the goods left behind. Both times this has happened to me (you would think I learned the first time!), both clients were 'fine' with it and, yes, I did see them again. Luckily this didn't happen to them again with me and they did become loyal clients after that.

I have to tell you that the first time it happened, I was fresh out of school and my knowledge of the waxing world was a bit vague. The second time it happened, I was overly confident—cocky you could maybe say—and was chatting too much. That is when the mishaps occur just as frequently as the times when your knowledge is vague. I knew if I had just sent them home, all waxed and bruised up without me apologizing, they would not have returned to me. Admitting you are wrong or that you have made a mistake is very difficult for some technicians or just people in general, but it's crucial to have excellent customer service when working in the service industry. It means that you have to be pretty humble and apologetic in your approach.

So, try to be humble and offer brilliant customer service when dealing with clients regardless of whether they are there for waxing or other services in your salon or spa. It calls for good etiquette and gets you more recognition in the long term. At the end of the day, who doesn't like to be treated fairly?

Let's recap. Keep the fingers under the tendon to avoid bruising around the upper thigh and always hold the skin taut when applying wax and removing wax. Doing this will always prevent bruising.

Incidentally if a client is on blood thinners, takes aspirin daily, or is vitamin deficient, then no matter what you do to prevent bruises during waxing they may still be more evident.

It is a funny thing about excellence. If you refuse to accept anything but the very best you often get it. W. Somerset Manghan

Tip 6: No Double Dipping

Never double dip! By this I mean that if you have stuck the spatula into the wax pot, then applied it to the area/ skin to be waxed, the stick should be thrown away in the trash can immediately. Imagine waxing every client with just one stick and you kept double dipping? The tin of wax would have traces of blood, pubic hair, and faeces (especially if the client didn't clean up properly!!). It would be a breeding ground for bacteria, which is extremely unsanitary and not fair on the clients. If you use small individual pots of wax for one client and one client only and throw the remains away, then, by all means, use just one stick. But, most tins come in standard sizes, and the waste and cost of throwing several wax tins away each day would be far more than the waste and cost of using lots of sticks.

Wax doesn't heat up to a high enough temperature to 'kill' any bacteria. This is a myth, so please don't be fooled into believing this. If anything, since it is kept at a warm temperature, it is more likely to be a perfect breeding ground for germs to fester and multiply. Germs love warm places! Sticks are inexpensive and it doesn't eat away at your profits. Increase your prices by a couple of dollars if it is a big financial concern to you and inform clients as to why your prices are slightly higher.

I would also strongly suggest that you place a sign in your room as well as on your menu or website, informing them that your policy is "no double dipping." Not all salons place signs as they just take it for granted clients know. I think this adds that 'extra' uniqueness to your services and business. Some clients wouldn't even think that this was an issue anyway as they may have been informed in the past by a previous aesthetician that the heat of the wax kills germs.

To save a bit of money on the sticks as you do go through a lot of them with body waxing, snap your sticks in half so you have two sticks for the price of one! I personally find the length of the half sticks not long enough though. I prefer a larger handle so I have less chance of getting wax on my gloves. As such, I am happy to just go through a lot of them, but if the waste is of concern to you, then you can try this method.

When I have dipped into the wax with one end of the stick and removed the hair, I then turn the stick around and, with one of the old muslin strips that I have used; I wrap it around the soiled end. I then use the clean side of the muslin as a handle and the other end to dip into the wax for the next application.

Some may point out that my gloved hands were on this stick prior to it touching the skin. In fact, my hands are on all the products that touch the client. Unless the State Board requires that I work in a NASA spacesuit, with mask and goggles, and spray myself and my client down every five minutes with anti-bacterial spray, then my method is what I shall do. I never double dip, and the used strip wrapped as a handle doesn't come into contact with the wax in the pot either.

It is clean and efficient. Even though money isn't necessarily or shouldn't be a big factor, the waste is really the bigger issue for me. I hate waste of any description and like to keep things recycled as much as possible. I also like to be as sanitary as possible, but I do draw the line at neurotic behaviour!

I will go into 'when it is ok to double dip' in the next chapter, if you still disagree with using hundreds of spatulas.

There are some fantastic waxing educators out there that don't follow this theory and have their own reasons for why it is ok to double dip. I will never criticize what they do or how they do it as that is not my style and it has never been proven from my research that it actually does cause cross contamination. This book is written so that I can share with you what I prefer to do and what I would like to receive if I was on the other end of the waxing service.

Tip 7: When it's Okay to Double Dip

Some technicians love to get their speed up so much so that they can see as many clients a day as possible. These are the technicians who find using new sticks instead of double dipping important but find that it can also be a bit time wasting. So, this is why I mention this method to you.

The method that I am suggesting may also be too time consuming unless you have a large four-heat wax heater since you do have to allow for each new fill of wax pellets to heat up. But, since the level of wax in the tin is low enough for only using on one client, it should heat up pretty quickly. If you can determine how much wax you will need for each client, this should work. And, I am sure over time and with lots of experience you will get some indication as to how much roughly you use. If a client is a regular of yours and you know what type of wax you use for them, then this can be heating up prior to their arrival, so you are not twiddling your thumbs waiting for their personal wax tin to heat up.

One idea is to buy Cirepil® wax pellets, which are little beads of wax that come in a jar or bags. If you keep some empty wax tins around, you can place an empty wax tin in your heater before each new client and fill it with as many beads you think you may need for just that "one" client. If that wax is to be used on just that one client alone then double dip to your heart's content.

Because the level of wax in the tin will be pretty low, please ensure, when heating it, that you allow for the low level of wax. By this I mean that if you keep it at the same temperature as you do for a full tin of wax, you may find it's too hot and you will need to wait for it to cool down. Remember, runny wax that drips very quickly in a steady stream off a spatula is too hot!

Just throw the tin away when you have finished waxing your client and use a new tin for each new client. Or, if you prefer, you can line a tin with foil and, when the wax has all gone, remove the foil and replace it with new foil in the tin for the next client. This way you are again avoiding waste and cutting down on cost.

Applying Hard Wax

Most of you are probably aware already from beauty school and prior training in waxing at your salon that hard wax is thicker in consistency and application and is removed without paper strips or muslin strips. Hard wax is fantastic for sensitive areas of the body, such as bikini areas, eyebrows, lips, etc. The reason for this is that hard wax, once applied correctly and at the right temperature, has less contact with the skin than soft wax due to its shrink wrap capabilities around the hair.

I always use hard wax on the scrotum (*and the labia when waxing the Lady Garden, due to its loose, soft texture*). I never use soft wax on the scrotum as I find the skin is too thin and loose. I do believe there are some technicians that do use soft wax in this area and they find it works for them and that is ok. I have sat in on a couple of classes where they used soft wax and I just winced the whole time!

I personally do not want to risk it and have a guy's scrotum split open on me or have him leaving my salon with traces of skin left behind as I think it is more likely to happen when using soft wax. So, unless your intention is to make handbags out of scrotum skin, stick to using hard wax!

Just as before when your client kept pulling his twig to keep the skin taut, your client should do the same thing with his scrotum. When you apply the wax in a certain area, he should pull his skin taut with both of his hands to help you with the application and removal of the wax.

Hard wax as discussed earlier is thicker than soft wax. When applying hard wax anywhere on the body a much firmer pressure is required. As you apply the wax you are actually "pressing" it down as if you are "pushing" it into the skin coating the base of the hair snuggly. Don't be afraid to press down as firm pressure when applying hard wax is the best way to get a great, clean result. By all means ask your client if the pressure is ok. If you pull the skin around your elbow, it really doesn't hurt. Try it. Pulling the skin on the scrotum or labia using your fingertips and not your nails doesn't hurt either and feels similar to the pressure when pulling on elbow skin. It is probably questionable as to whether it hurts or not if your fingernails resemble Freddie Krueger. If that is the case, keep them short!

As you work around the sides of his scrotum going from the inside of his thigh to the centre of the scrotum, he pulls the skin away from you. His scrotum is like a bean bag and moves around easily, hence the reason he should help you by keeping it out of your way.

If you applied hard wax onto a floppy bean bag and then let it loose, the bean bag with wax applied to it would flop against the bean bag that didn't have wax applied to it and it might stick. So apply a light dusting of powder over the freshly applied wax rather than waiting for it to dry, to avoid it sticking to other parts of the body.

I work my way around his scrotum, starting on one side, and then moving over to the other side. Once both sides are clean, I then work on the middle section of his scrotum. Again, when working on the middle section, I check the direction of hair growth and apply the wax accordingly all the while, whilst he pulls the skin away from where I am working.

Some people like to use a tiny amount of oil prior to the skin before waxing. Depending on the skin and the client's hair, I either use oil or powder. Sometimes I like to use powder more as it shows up the difficult to see hairs, which helps me! I prefer to powder up the scrotum, so that he has an easier grip on the skin whilst he is pulling. If oil is applied, he finds it harder to grip the skin while he is keeping it stretched for you.

When you go down under to apply the wax on his perineum (the space between his bum crack and the base of his scrotum) have him pull his sack upwards with both hands towards his belly with his legs slightly spread like a frog. This allows you to get in there easily and again keeps the skin taut. Powder up the area; apply the wax and using a removal method of your choice remove the wax.

If the hair is growing upwards in this area as is usually the case, when you remove the wax keeping it parallel to the skin as usual, you will find that you may punch the massage bed as you are so close to it.

Sometimes if my client isn't heavy set, I get him to raise his hips off the bed slightly, so I have more room to remove the wax. If you feel you are left with very little space to remove this section of wax, you have a tendency to 'flick' the wax off, instead of removing it parallel as you are conscious of the bed getting in the way of your hand motion. When we flick wax off as opposed to removing it parallel, it doesn't make for a clean finish, it breaks the hair off, leaving traces of stubble behind. I go into different methods of hard wax removal in tips nine and ten.

Hard wax should always be pretty close to body temperature. If it is runny and drips off the spatula, it is way too hot and should be left to cool down by leaving the lid off the pot and turning the temperature knob down. One of my favourite hard waxes is Cirepil® Blue from France. It has a lovely aroma with a great consistency to it. Generally Cirepil® should be used with oil rather than powder. If the powder is used "sparingly" I still find that I get a great application and result. I like the majority of their waxes, but this one has to be my favourite of all time. (No, I am not on commission with Cirepil®. I just like to share with people what I love and what has worked for me).

Once the wax is applied to the hair, it causes a shrink-wrap effect around the hair, making for easier removal. Hard wax sticks to the hair and not to the skin per se. The beauty of using this wax is that it can be applied in the same area more than once.

I am not saying to keep going over and over the same area hundreds of times, but you have much less chance of burning or lifting the skin than if you did this with soft wax. I do try to avoid applying even hard wax over the same area twice, especially on the scrotum. I just hope my application and correct method of removal is sufficient enough the first time to avoid going over the same area a second time.

But generally, hard wax is pretty much safe to wax over the same area more than once. This is true except if the temperature is way too hot and you burn the living daylights out of him. I am sure this won't happen as we have already discussed the correct consistency and temperature of the wax prior to applying it to the skin.

If you do happen to go over the same area more than once with the hard wax, due to the skin's sensitivity at already receiving wax in this area, the temperature of the wax applied should be cooler, so as not to alert your client with the increase of heat or to burn him.

Reach into the tin with your clean spatula taking the wax from the top without scraping the barrel at the bottom and then keep the wax on the spatula a bit longer, to allow it to cool, before applying it. I have seen some technicians blow the wax like they are spoon feeding their child—there is something about blowing on a waxing spatula that I just find unprofessional!

I have been taught a few different ways of how to apply hard wax. I was taught my favourite way in England, again by my wonderful teacher! I have also heard from a couple of people that wax should never be applied by fudging or by double-siding the hair due to breakage. I have never found this to be the case and I consistently get good results doing it this way.

So, next I will share with you the technique that has always worked well for me. This way, you can try it and see if you like it too. You may want to stick with the regular rule of always applying hard wax towards the hair growth. Again, it's whatever works for you.

Tip 8: Another Way of Applying Hard Wax

At this point, hopefully, he still has some dusted powder or a tiny bit of oil around the base of his twig so hard wax can be applied. If he doesn't, apply a little bit more to protect the skin. Again, using a clean spatula so no double dipping occurs, plunge the spatula into the tin from the side, making sure you have a nice fair amount on the end of the spatula like a big garlic bulb.

Sometimes, when pulling the spatula away from the tin with the wax attached to the end, there are 'stringy' bits of wax attached to it. I have seen some aestheticians keep pulling the spatula away from the tin to help detach the strings, but then they spun themselves around in circles or, even worse, circle the spatula above their head trying to get rid of the stringy wax. The result is that they then became like a cocoon of blue wax where it sticks to their clothes, the equipment, the walls and even their shoes!

If you have done this, I am sure you will be smiling right now as you know exactly what I am talking about! With the spatula and blob of wax attached to the end, just waft it back and forth in the tin very close to the heat of the wax without actually touching the wax in the tin, and this will break the string free for you. Incidentally, when you have applied the hard wax onto the body, waft the spatula back and forth, close to the wax application also. The heat from the wax will prevent strings.

The wax is then applied *firmly* in a figure of eight. Apply the wax going down the hair in a section *towards* the hair growth, then back up again and around and up the hair *against* the hair growth, then completing the circuit again by going back *towards* the hair growth. In this way, you are forming a figure eight in one of your sections, which will be about 1 ½"—2" in width and length. What this does is coat the hair on both sides.

When you apply the wax, always try to keep the edges of the wax around the figure eight in an even consistency. When some of the edges are too thin, as they dry, they then become brittle. When pulled off the skin, this tends to leave annoying traces of hard wax. Leave the wax to dry for a couple of minutes and, whilst you are doing this, you can prepare your hard wax removal handle.

I can explain another way of applying the hard wax if you are not happy with the figure eight method. Basically, the wax is applied using a clean spatula again onto the hair in the direction of the hair growth just the same as applying soft wax. Again, keep the edges the same thickness so it doesn't get too thin. A lip can be formed or you can use another method of removal using a handle of your choice. The wax is applied in the direction of hair growth and removed against it. It is removed by keeping it as close to the skin as possible just like when waxing with soft wax.

This is quite simple with no fuss and the best part of all is that you don't need to be a rocket scientist to figure it out. But, for some reason I just find this way doesn't get as 'clean' a result as what I would like hence the reason I prefer the figure 8 method. However, you may love to apply it this way and want to stick with it. Whatever works for you safely and for your client is the way you should go and the way you should stick to. Be comfortable, but be safe.

When the smooth get testy, the testes get smooth!

Tip 9: Removing Hard Wax

U sing a clean spatula, dip into the tin, remove a blob of wax from the side about the size of a quarter coin, and blob the wax onto the inside of your arm where there is no hair. To speed up the drying process, sprinkle some powder over it and dab it lightly. Sprinkling powder onto hard wax speeds up the drying time.

When the figure of eight is firm to the touch and ready to remove, you can then take the dried blob that is sitting on the inside of your arm and, with the shiny side of the wax (the wax that is not touching your arm), form a tab onto the figure eight to work as your handle. Place the wax from the inside of your arm onto the wax where you want to lift it from and remove the wax from your client this way. Think shiny side to dull side.

Lift the wax from the hair against the hair growth, using your wax handle to remove it. The reason I use a handle is to prevent picking at the edges of the wax, which can sometimes cause more discomfort than the wax removal itself. So, don't pick at the edges to remove it, use a handle or leave a larger blob of wax for easy removal as explained below.

Picking at the edges of the wax bugs the "geebies" out of people and feels very irritating, inevitably also picking at their skin. The scrotum is super thin so this isn't advisable!

Removing hard wax is the same principle as removing soft wax. Pull it away from the hair/skin as parallel to the body as possible to prevent leaving traces of hair or breaking it off at the surface.

Another way of removing hard wax is by making a much thicker blob of wax in the area where you know you want to remove the wax from. This is called 'forming a lip.' The area left will be thicker and with a slight lip at the side and this can also be used as your handle when removing the wax to again avoid picking.

Tip 10: Daisy Chain

Another way of removing the hard wax is to create what I call a Daisy Chain or a Caterpillar Trail. This is an advanced method that is used once your technique is up to speed and you are pretty confident with your waxing services. Now your brain might be buzzing around like a fly in a shoe box taunted by the different removal methods, but they are all actually good tips to have up your sleeve and make your business much more fun and effective.

So, now Mr. Client has a figure eight of wax stuck to his "wotsits" and you are waiting for it to dry. This isn't the only hair around his scrotum or his pubic regions so once you have applied this section with hard wax go onto another section and do the same thing again. This can be done three or four times in different sections around the area, coating different sections of hair.

When you look at his nether regions, you will see that he has patches of wax all over him in different places. This method is used in speed waxing and, again, I wouldn't do this method until you are pretty confident with your technique. You also have to have a pretty good memory as to which section you did first, which section has hair growing in what direction, etc. so you know from what direction the wax needs to be removed from and know that one patch hasn't been sitting on there forever, going all brittle like hard candy.

With practice and knowing your (N, E, S, W) rule of thumb, it starts to become second nature. Let's say for argument sake you have four sections of wax scattered around his "wotsits." The first section by now will be pretty dry so you remove this first section (by using a handle of your choice). With the shiny side of the wax that you have *just* removed, attach it to section number two and pull the second section off using the first blob of wax as your handle. Keep, using these as your wax handles until all waxed sections have been removed. It makes the removal process much quicker and you avoid picking at the wax. Again, think shiny side to dull side.

Tip 11: Positions

Everything above is super smooth—no hickies, no irritated skin, and a happy smiley client. Now it's time to get the client to turn over so you can wax his bum crack.

There are four different ways that I have been taught how to do this. Anatomy of the client does play a big part in how we wax this area as does the client's personality.

Each of the four ways is explained below. You can be the judge of what you like the best and I will share with you what I do prefer and why.

1. The cannonball position
   With your client lying on his back, ask him to bring his knees up to his chest, spreading his legs slightly as he does this. He will resemble a trussed up turkey ready for roasting without the little white caps on his feet! Please note that this is not an easy position for a heavy set client to get into.

   Once he is in this position, you can get a good view of his bum obviously, but it also forces the area to be waxed to be pulled pretty taut, which makes application and removal easier.

He also has a much higher chance of breaking wind whilst he is in this position and, personally, I don't want to be on the receiving end of it! I am not a lover of this position for my clients, or for myself.

Apply the powder to his exposed area so the powder sticks to the hair and not so much his bum hole. Apply the hard wax in small sections and, once dry, remove the wax.

Strangely enough, all clients tell me that this area is not at all painful, but actually feels quite nice to have the warm wax applied here and then removed. I ask no questions about their private life or their fetish that involves hot wax applied to their bum. To each their own is my philosophy. After all, what do I care what they find soothing in the comfort of their own home!

2. <u>Doggy Style position</u>
    Get your client to get on all fours on the bed, again with his legs spread slightly apart. You will have to get him to spread one bum cheek apart with one hand whilst balancing on the bed with his other hand to support him. This is not an easy task for an older client or a very heavy client. The visual is also not a good one and will stay inputted in your brain for many months to come!

    The bum cheek that is spread apart makes it easy for you to apply the powder and the wax because the skin is taut so it makes it easier. Encourage him to pull tightly to keep the skin as taut as possible. Of course, you can also pull one bum cheek apart, whilst you apply and remove the wax. It's whatever you find the easiest.

3. Flat Waxley

   Get your client to lie down on the massage bed onto his stomach. Then have him spread both of his bum cheeks apart as wide as possible to make applying powder and the wax as well as the removal easier. Prep the skin and apply the wax as normal. This is my favourite position for clients to be in. I feel they have some dignity left and have less chance of breaking wind (which is enough of a reason to prefer this position). It is also a pretty standard easy position for any client regardless of body shape, type, etc.

4. Side Plank.

   This position is very similar to Flat Waxley but with the client lying on his side. I like this way of doing it also, especially if the client is slightly claustrophobic and doesn't like his face pressed into the bed or massage/facial hole. This is the way that most midwives remove stitches following child birth. It also allows the client to keep some dignity as they feel less exposed. He will still need to help by pulling his bum cheek slightly apart so that you can get into the area easily with your wax and will also keep the skin taut, making removal much easier.

Excellence is not a skill. It is an attitude.
Ralph Marston.

Client Clean-Up

Check under your magnifying light for any stray hairs that hopefully you didn't miss! If you really have to, get out the tweezers and tweeze away at a few of them. This should not be a big part of the clean up process and, with practice and experience; the tweezers shouldn't be used very much.

This is also a time during the clean up process where you will see if (god forbid!) any skin has lifted. What you will see if this has happened is a change in texture on the skin. It will have a 'shine' to the skin. This 'shine' to the skin is what will scab over and cause discomfort to the client. It is basically new skin and I hope this doesn't happen to you, but if it does, apply a small amount of Neosporin® and tell your client apologetically that unfortunately this has happened and that he will need to continue dabbing it to the area once he is home for the next few days.

No matter how wonderful a soothing lotion is like the one I mention below, I would advise against using it over these lifted patches of skin as it can sting! But hopefully, we have no lifted skin and he just has minor discomfort without major stinging and we can lavish him with lotion instead.

A great product to use on your client during the clean-up process is Res-Q™ by Satin Smooth™. It is an analgesic soothing cream with 4% Lidocaine in it, which quickly relieves temporary minor skin irritation and numbs the skin very slightly.

I actually apply this before I begin the tweezing so it makes the tweezing less irritating as it numbs the skin slightly. Most clients do tell me that they find it really does numb the prickly sensation left from the waxing. Unfortunately, it does say on the box that this product cannot be used prior to waxing.

It is a great product to retail also. Send him home with a tube of it and get him to use it once he is home following every waxing service with you. This product is also one of my favourites to use after I have done an eyebrow wax. Clients absolutely love the gentle brow massage I give to them when using it!

With your client holding himself like a joy stick again, apply a nice Aloe Vera soothing lotion, hydrocortisone lotion, salicylic acid 1% or 2% lotion or any other nice soothing lotion by the company of your choice. Rub the lotion into your gloved hands to warm it up a little bit and to help with the slick. I like to use Clean and Easy® Restore (it's the only one that I have ever used and was happy with the slickness of it and have never strayed from using it).

Apply the lotion, rubbing it in gently, but efficiently. I say efficiently as the soothing motions and gentle stroking as you rub down there is not fair on the poor guy and takes your professionalism to a gutter level.

If he has some sticky residue left from waxing on his twig, get him to rub around that area to help remove it. Those soothing orgasmic sounds a client makes when you give him a nice back rub with your lotions and potions following a back wax are okay and you feel a sense of pride as you know you are making him feel better. But, I don't feel comfortable hearing those sounds from his pie hole when I am down under. So keep the clean up process efficient and professional.

I would not recommend handing him a hot towel at this point to soothe his nether regions as the area is delicate and probably a bit red from the waxing. At this point, a slight amount of redness is perfectly normal. However, red skin and hot towels are not a good combination. Wait for the damp towel to reach a comfortable temperature before applying it to the area to help relieve some irritation and to calm the skin down.

During the clean-up period, this may be a good time (if you have the time on your books) to cross-sell your services. If you noticed whilst you were waxing him that he had hair on his back or his chest, then by all means ask him if this is a concern for him. If he is happy with his back/chest hair, then don't push it by suggesting he needs to have it removed as you may be getting too personal. His partner may like the cuddly teddy bear look, BUT chances are he/she won't, especially if he is in for waxing his nether regions. If he shows some interest, then inform him that you have time today to clean that area up for him. If he doesn't have time that day, suggest it for his next visit.

This is also a good time to suggest to him that it is important to keep on as much as a schedule as possible and become a regular at waxing to maintain the hair growth. If he shaves in between, the hair will grow back coarser; making his next wax feel like it is his first wax and really defeats the object of waxing.

Hair grows back finer the more that you wax it. Some of the follicles die or weaken, causing the hair to grow back slightly sparser and fluffier than if they were to shave or to use depilatory creams. Clients do find that it gets easier with each wax that they have due to this very reason.

Unfortunately it never gets to the point of no hair growth as this doesn't happen with waxing! Explaining to them the reasons behind why waxing is so beneficial also helps them to understand why they put themselves through the whole procedure!

Inform him that every four weeks is a good period, but this can vary with each client and can also vary due to different ethnic backgrounds. Some clients may need waxing every six weeks as opposed to four. Or if you want to suggest to him that he follows the "Ideal" waxing procedure as discussed earlier you could do this also.

There are a couple of things that your client needs to know before he leaves your salon. Advise him to avoid Jacuzzi's, tanning beds, sauna's or steam rooms for at least 24 hours following a wax. The pores have been opened and are more prone to infection. Going to the gym *immediately* following a wax is also not advisable, as sweat can cause the skin to break out or become irritated.

A nice warm tepid shower with nothing too scented or abrasive for 24 hours is the best way to treat the areas that have been waxed. After 24 hours, if the skin is not too inflamed or generally irritated then to help prevent in-grown hairs a good sugar scrub is great to use twice a week followed by a good soothing lotion to keep the skin calm in the nether regions.

As mentioned earlier in the book I would not recommend using a Loofah due to its porous nature and ability to harbour yeast!

I like to tell my clients that their skin has been through some sort of minor trauma and to treat it, just like they would if they had sunburn. After all you wouldn't go rubbing yourself with an abrasive scrub, steaming yourself like a vegetable or tanning your body, if you were already sunburnt!

Wearing tight fitting jeans is ok if they have had a wax from the waist up, but anything below the waist, then they need to wear loose, comfortable fitting clothes for at least 24 hours. This helps prevent chaffing of the skin and also helps prevent in-grown hairs!

Some clients may break out regardless of your skill or which wax was used. If this is the case it is best that they come back in to see you so that you can inspect their area of concern and recommend a product to help them with this. Witch Hazel is a great inexpensive product to use at home if they break out or suffer from any irritation. A good homemade mix whipped up in the kitchen of aspirin and water is a good topical treatment to use also to help with any irritation. If possible, let them know that breakouts sometimes happen and that 'next time' you will use a wax specifically for sensitive skin. If it is their very first wax appointment, then let them know this is very common and it sometimes takes a few sessions for their skin to get used to it.

If this does happen to one of your clients then make a note of it on their client record card: so you can either, ask them about it again the next time you see them or call them to find out how they are doing, if you haven't seen them for a while.

This shows that you took the time to remember their issue that they had with their last waxing appointment and again that you care!

How to Remove Ingrown Hairs

Ingrown hairs are very common in the bikini area. They are generally caused by incorrect waxing, or shaving. They are also caused by wearing very tight, synthetic underwear or tight jeans following a wax. When the skin isn't allowed to breathe it sweats and bacteria gets trapped leading to zits and ingrown hairs.

Exfoliating the area twice a week with a nice scrub, helps unclog the pores by removing the dead skin cells surrounding the follicle.

Using a nice hot compress applied to the area for five minutes will help draw out the gunk making its exit strategy easier. Gently apply pressure either side of the bump where the ingrown hair is to see if this helps. If nothing seems to be coming out, apply your hot compress again and repeat the process.

If you still have no joy, then leave it alone. Too much squeezing can rupture the follicle underneath the skin resulting in an infection, bleeding or scarring.

If you do see the tip of the hair pop out when applying pressure to the area—using your clean, sanitized pointy tweezers remove the hair and then apply a Tea Tree astringent compress to help remove any bacteria. Tea Tree has wonderful properties as its natural agent cures fungus, bacteria and most viruses. It can also be used as a mouthwash diluted with water if you have forgotten your toothbrush!

If it still looks slightly inflamed a touch of high frequency will help reduce the inflammation and help to kill any bacteria that may be present. Even better to help with reducing inflammation and the extraction of an ingrown hair is Epsom salts.

Epsom salts are named from a bitter, saline spring at Epsom in Surrey, England. It is not actually a salt but a natural occurring mineral with 'amazing' health benefits which contain magnesium and sulphites. These two powerful ingredients help remove ingrown hairs as they are both readily absorbed through the skin improving the absorption of nutrients and aid in flushing out the toxins. The salts when used as a compress alleviate pain and inflammation. It also exfoliates the dead skin cells without causing a stinging sensation. It is a great alternative from using just a regular compress of hot water. Epsom salts are very, very inexpensive and can be found in any pharmacy in the U.S.A. They can be used for a whole variety of ailments and not just for the flushing out of ingrown hairs. Buy a large, medicine glass bottle and store your labelled salts in there, to use in your salon for cleaning, medicinal purposes or to just look 'fancy'!

Mix 2 tablespoons of Epsom salt into a bowl with 8 oz of distilled water (tap water is ok, but it's preferable to use distilled) Soak your cotton compress into the solution and leave on the infected or ingrown area for a minimum of ten minutes.

Epsom salts rough texture makes it an ideal exfoliator which you can use on yourself at home. Massage handfuls of it over your body during your shower to rid the skin of any dead skin cells and to give you that healthy, happy glow! It can also be mixed in with a cleanser as a facial scrub. Tea Tree can be added to your little mixture too, if you have oily skin.

You can tell your clients about this wonderful alternative to an expensive scrub, but if retail is where you make most of your profits, maybe you can keep this secret to yourself!

Tip 12: High Frequency

A little device that so many of my male clients love is the high frequency machine. Whenever I wax a client's back or chest and he appears to be on the red side or is prone to breaking out, I get out the ole faithful high frequency machine.

High frequency kills bacteria, speeds up the healing process, and the current from the high frequency provides an infusion of oxygen molecules into his skin. The high frequency current also produces a cleaning and massaging method. The massage stimulates the blood flow, which helps carry the waste away by the lymphatic system. The client will experience a therapeutic tingling sensation and for some reason makes men feel ever so loved!!

It is also nice to use around the brow area if your client is heading back into work after an eyebrow wax. Apply the Res-Q™ to the area that has been waxed. Then give a nice soothing brow massage applying gentle pressure to the brow bone and then apply the High frequency. It also helps to reduce the redness and again makes them feel that you are taking extra care into their needs. Avoid the eyeballs; just glide it across the brow bone for a minute or so!

I like to use this machine when I have waxed his twigs and berries also. I glide it over the skin with the Res-Q™ cream and facial gauze on the area and again, I inform him why I am doing this. Believe me, if for some reason my machine is broken and in for repair, I literally get the pout from the client and he feels put out that he hasn't had a little bit of loving. He literally leaves the building with his shoulders hunched over that he hasn't had this, but smiles like a Cheshire cat when he has received it. Be smart and have two machines. There's nothing worse than a pouting man!

If like I mentioned earlier he has some lifted skin (God forbid!) then the high frequency applied over the area with the Neosporin® and facial gauze on it will help with the healing process also.

Remember when applying the high frequency machine to keep your finger on the glass mushroom probe until it touches the skin. If you place the glass probe directly to the skin without easing your finger off it when you touch him, it will spark and shock him. It will not shock him as in giving him an electric shock or by hurting him, but it will just startle him as it will feel like a rubber band twanging against his nether regions. So, remember, each time you remove the probe or apply the probe, keep the pointer finger on it until contact is made.

Clients really do like it, and it does reduce a lot of the redness and is very beneficial for zits and the prevention of further breakouts, but it is also soothing to the skin due to its oxygenating properties. All these benefits surely help towards increasing your retention rate and tips!

However, those clients who are epileptic or who have a pacemaker are not a good candidate for this machine. So, if you plan on using a high frequency machine after waxing, ask your clients if they are epileptic or have a pacemaker.

In normal brain function we have millions of tiny electrical charges that pass from our nerve cells in the brain to the rest of the body. When the brain function is interrupted by unusual bursts of electrical energy (which high frequency produces) a person who is epileptic receiving this may have a reaction, resulting in a seizure.

Pacemaker failures can occur when they are exposed to high voltage electricity. High frequency interferes with their device and can be fatal.

Clients with metal implants are also advised not to use high frequency. Exposure to rapidly changing magnetic fields on metal implants can cause parts of the body to heat up. A decisive factor is the conductivity of the metal. Heat that is produced is conducted to the surrounding tissue and in a worst case scenario can cause the surrounding tissue to sustain burns.

Room Preparation

Your client has just left and you are getting ready for your next client to show. Hopefully, you have a 15 minute window where you have sufficient time to clean your room, once the product sales have closed and the niceties are out of the way.

Don't let your idea of housekeeping be 'sweeping' the room with a glance, as housekeeping is something you do that nobody notices, until you *don't* do it!

Remove all sheets and towels used during your last clients visit and dispose of them in the laundry basket. Incidentally all towels and sheets should be washed on a 40°C hot cycle and dried on "high" in the dryer.

All disposable items like spatula's, strips, paper sheeting and gloves should be thrown away immediately so you can begin to wipe down your area ready for the next client to arrive.

Tweezers should be washed with hot soapy water, dried and then immersed in a jar of Barbicide®. Your tweezers should be immersed for a minimum of ten minutes. This product does have an anti-rust formula, so if you leave them in for longer you will not have ruined tweezers.

Barbicide® is a U.S.A, EPA registered, hospital grade, broad spectrum disinfectant. It is a Germicide, Pseudomonacide, fungicide and virucide. It kills pseudomonas, staph and salmonella. Original Barbicide® also kills HIV—1 (AIDS virus) Hepatitis B and Hepatitis C on pre-cleaned surfaces and objects previously soiled with blood and bodily fluids.

Wash your hands and begin to prep your room for your next client. Place clean sheets and towels on the bed and set up your table with a clean towel or paper towel ready for your next client. If the paper collar around your waxing pot is very heavily soiled, I would advise you to throw this away and replace with a new one.

If you needed to use the clippers on your client and find that you have tumbleweeds of hair on your tiled floor, starting to resemble a finely crafted rug, sweep up around your area, leaving the floor clean. I specifically mentioned "tiled" floor as carpeting in a waxing room is not advisable due to sanitation and in most states it is against State Board regulations.

If you have a very busy schedule with back to back clients, you may find it easier to layer your bed like a Lasagne! You can drape the bed with a sheet, a towel, then another sheet, a towel and keep adding to the bed draping. This helps to save you on time and a lot of Spa's in high end hotels do this when they have back to back facials or massages.

After each client leaves, remove the sheet and towel that they were laying on and the fresh linens will be on the bed all ready for the next client. This does save time, especially if your linen cupboard isn't in your room but down the corridor.

Some salons that like to save money on the utility bills are happy to just 'flip' the sheets and towels over ready for the next client. Please, don't do this. It isn't very sanitary; also sweaty "Eau De Towel" smell isn't appealing to the nose.

Claire's Favourite Picks

I choose these as my favourite products as they have served me well.

I am not on commission from any of the companies that I mention below or in any part of this book. And, I don't mention any other products out there on the market that may do as 'just a good job' as I have never tried them so I cannot comment on them. There are some products out there that I have been told about very recently that are also fantastic, but, for now, I will share with you the one's that have worked for me in the past.

- Cirepil® Ocean Blue
- Cirepil® Blue
- Cirepil® Blanche
- Cirepil® Pearl
- Cirepil® Skin Prep Oil
- Cirepil® Cristal Cleansing Lotion
- Satin Smooth Res-Q™
- Gigi® Anaesthetic Numbing Spray
- Clean and Easy Restore®
- Epsom salts
- Tea Tree

These are available from most professional beauty supply stores or online.

If anybody is looking for good recommendations on waxing experts in the U.S.A you can find classes/materials at www.premierbeautysolutions.com

The Art of Sales

"Sales", is not a dirty word! Some technicians cringe when they think of the word, "Sales." Try and erase that word from your vocabulary. If it makes it easier use the word "consult" if that rings better with you. We all think of used car salesmen with cheesy slicked back hair and a plaid suit when we think of sales, but it doesn't have to be that way.

Whenever you are consulting with a client about what you are doing, what products you are using and why you are using them, in effect you are selling to them simply by educating them. When you inform them that you offer other services in your salon, inform them by making polite conversation that you offer this. Again, this is essentially selling. Listen to what your clients tell you and how they respond.

Don't just presume that because you think you have the best aftercare lotion or offer the best facial in town that they are in a position right now to buy. Advise your clients as to why you think they "need" the product or the service and how it would "benefit" them. Don't push; just consult with them as to why it could potentially be beneficial to them.

The same goes with cross-selling services. If you casually mention, "Hey I have 30 minutes to kill before my next client. If your back hair bothers you, we could wax that for you today to save you another visit." Again, don't just presume that his back hair does bother him as you could insult him. You will get lot's of "Sorry, not right now", *or* "Maybe next time I will try it" *or* "Hmm, let me think about it" Don't take it personally when a client say's no to you. If you are truly authentic and consult from the heart this will soon become evident and trust will soon be built.

I once went into a spa that came highly recommended for a skin consultation as I was just looking for a nice aromatic relaxing facial. We were happily sat chatting about this for a good 10 minutes and I was warming up to her and ready to schedule my future relaxing Vitamin C facial appointment. But, then she squinted her eyes at my forehead, twisted her nose as if she disapproved, and suggested I get the wrinkles on my forehead dealt with, by booking in for some Botox also!! She was thinking money and I was thinking, "Rude!!" She didn't listen to a word I said and, at the same time, she 'presumed' that because my poor wrinkles offended her that they offended me also. I felt insulted so my wrinkly forehead and I left her consultation room (head bowed down in shame) without so much as a future appointment or a recommendation from me!

The point I am trying to make is remember the rule: "You have two ears and one mouth for a reason!

When you are cleaning the client and using the numbing lotion or talking to him about the sugar scrub, tell him why you are using it or why it would benefit him before or after each appointment and that it would be a great take home product for him to buy so that he has it there ready for his next appointment to use. When you walk him out to reception area, leave the product on the counter, again show him what you are recommending he buys today, and if he has any questions, you are there to answer them. If you don't show him the product that you are suggesting, he could potentially walk right out of your door to the local pharmacy and buy from them instead, or buy a product that is not appropriate for his skin type.

Send out 'thank you' cards if they are a new client. Keep it professional and not cutesy, the last thing you want is some suspicious crazy, rabbit boiling partner to steam into your location or to accuse him at home of inappropriate behaviour. I once worked with a girl who sent out a thank you card to a first time client. She wrote on the card "Was so nice seeing you last week, looking forward to the next time". His girlfriend found the card in his car and consequently a fight broke out, he was in the dog house for a week and he never returned to the salon again, but did call us to explain the reason about why he wouldn't be returning! So, keep it very professional and not cutesy. Everything you write should be written as if it will be read by a partner of the client.

Keep a cheat sheet on that client with things that they have told you—maybe their dog's name, or their children's names, etc. So, when they return, you can look back at your cheat sheet and ask them about their dog, "Ruffus" or how little "Willy" did in his piano recital. People love to be remembered. If you do this often enough, it will soon be lodged into your brain about this persons personal life and you won't need to keep referring back to your cheat sheet . . . unless of course they are updating you on a vacation that they are about to take. Ask them about it when you see them again. It really makes a difference to that person's experience when you show that you care and that you have listened.

Ask them if they would like to be on your mailing list, so that you can keep them posted about special offers, etc. If they have supplied you with their email address on the consultation form, don't just presume that you can bombard them with your newsletters. Ask them first if they would like to receive them. They may say 'no' in which case just use the email as a confirmation use only. Once your client has agreed to receiving newsletters, make sure that you have an "Unsubscribe" option on the bottom of it, so they can at any time decide if it's not for them. I am actually very surprised as to how many companies I receive newsletters from that don't have this unsubscribe option. I find it very annoying.

Mention that he will receive a confirmation call the day before his appointment and possibly a confirmation email also. He may have a preference whether it is phone or email. Listen to what he prefers and use the method he is asking for.

This is also a fantastic time to say, "It was lovely seeing you today. Thank you so much for coming to see me. It is always appreciated and I will see you in four/six weeks time for your next appointment." He will know why you find it important to see him in this time frame as during the clean up you will have told him why. Shake his hand (as remember shaking hands in business at the end of a service shows that you are grateful for his business), smile nicely, and thank him again. Try and keep at least 15 minutes between each client, to allow for clean up time, sales, and friendly goodbyes!

As a final motivator, remember it's cheaper and easier to keep your existing clients than to find new ones. Therefore, the more clients that return the more productive and profitable your salon will be.

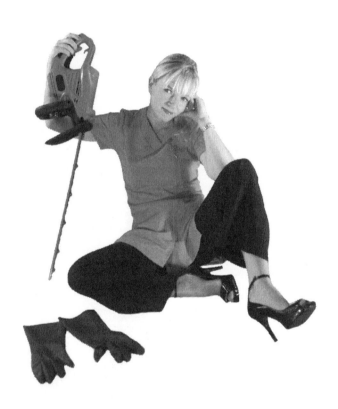

Rewards Programs

Does your Salon or Spa offer them? Rewards programs are a great way to keep your customers happy and coming back and talking about your place to other people. Some people are so busy focusing on getting new clients that they forget their existing ones. So try some of these reward programs to see what works best for you.

Before he leaves, tell him about the rewards program that you have going on in your salon. For every time he re-books an appointment and keeps that appointment, he can receive 10% off of his next visit. He can call and change the appointment to another date or time and still get the discount. But, if he cancels with the intention of calling back another day to schedule, then unfortunately he loses the discount. With him knowing this, he is more likely to reschedule there and then on the phone and stick with the appointment.

Give out a handful of your business cards with 'his' name written on the back. For every new client that comes to see you with the business card in hand, and his name on the back of it, he then receives a discount for taking the time out and recommending his friends and family to you. His friends who come in with the business card can also leave with more cards with their name on the back of them also, so that they can also recommend you to their friends and family. It doesn't have to be just for a waxing service; you could offer it for any service that you are licensed or certified to perform.

If they upgrade their services or try new services, use this as part of the rewards program also. They gain a point for every time they try something new or upgrade. These points can be accumulated over a year. Perhaps they gain five points for referring a friend, or two points for trying a new service etc. At some point once they have collected enough points, which equates to dollars, they could potentially get a service for free! Offering little incentives or reward programs make people feel special. Who doesn't like to be made to feel special?

If your client is a regular who spends a juicy amount of money with you each year, reward them with becoming a silver, gold or platinum member all depending on the dollar amount that they have spent with you each year. With each level that they reach they get discounts or a free hand massage, or free product. The higher the level they reach, the better the reward.

Another option is to give free movie tickets to the client who referred somebody to you. By giving a pair of tickets to your client when he takes his partner to the movies, their partner will know where the tickets came from, so you will have created another word-of-mouth machine.

If you are cost conscious like we all are these days check with your local cinema to buy a pack of tickets at a discount so you are not paying full face value.

Most clients don't expect anything, but are very happily surprised when they do receive something. Again you are becoming memorable and irreplaceable.

Social Media

I strongly recommend you use social media as one of your marketing tools. By social media, I mean using Twitter and Facebook. These tools are a great way for you to post updates to your fans or followers about any special offers that your salon may have or any updates about new staff members coming on board. What social media is NOT is a place for you to just sell, sell, and sell. If used correctly, it can greatly increase your profits and credibility.

When using social media as your marketing tool, you are still accountable for keeping your branding alive. You still have a store front at your salon/spa where you engage with clients and people who walk through your door. When people walk through your door at your location, you hopefully show an interest in them while they are visiting. So, sometimes I am left scratching my head as to why people who use social media as their marketing tool ignore their fans or followers.

Engage, engage, and engage. Ask your followers on your chosen social media site questions and respond to their replies. Maybe you could ask them about their favourite holiday or hobby. It is all about building relationships and showing that you care about them.

With Twitter, you need to tweet consistently to create momentum. Since there is a steady stream of tweets, your tweet can get lost in the active flow of twitters! Twitter is referred to as a cocktail party. Jump in and join conversations. If you find somebody has tweeted something that you find interesting, re-tweet what they have said to your followers. When people comment on your tweets or re-tweet something wonderful that you have announced, 'thank' them. Don't ignore them. Remember, if they came into your salon, would you ignore them?

Again, don't just sell, sell, sell or you may lose your followers and become a bit of a bore. We don't want face-ache nor do we want to appear as a twit-face! Be authentic and post good content that keeps people engaged. When I log onto Twitter and up pops a tweet from a person that I recognize, I smile. I don't always get that feeling if it is a picture of their company logo. I just associate the logo with the person trying to sell me something. What makes me feel all fuzzy and wuzzy inside is a person who wants to build relationships with me and cares about me as their potential client.

Twitter has different ways of allowing you to tweet. They have applications like "HootSuite" and many more that allow you to schedule tweets ahead of time. This can save time, but remember to periodically change your scheduled tweets so it stays authentic and doesn't make you appear like a robot or a spam bot.

Facebook is slightly different as your comments; and status stays on the page until you delete it and it doesn't get lost in the flow like it can do on Twitter. Incidentally, don't use your personal/friend page as your business Facebook. Use a business Facebook page and keep it strictly for clients or potential clients. The last thing you need is clients seeing posted pictures of you swinging from a chandelier flashing your knickers off to the cyber world during a night out with the girls in Vegas!

I still think it is great to post good content, ask your fans questions, and respond back to their posts. Post updates about special offers that you have, but don't just use this as your only way of interacting. Occasionally, post a comment about how grateful you are for your fans and how you value them. Update your page daily and be sure to keep it short but sweet.

Check out your local library or book store for books/e-books on social media. Stay ahead of the game and keep up-to-date with newer methods of marketing. This is the future so flyers are pretty much a thing of the past!

Social Media is a great tool for marketing. It is also a great tool for employers to investigate their staff, or new hires. Prior to an interview, make sure your social media sites reflect a professional image of yourself. Some potential employers might check up on you, to see if your profile fits what you have told them in the interview. I do know of some business owners who have done a quick check on potential hires through social media sites. It helps them with the decision making process after an interview. If you don't know what is appropriate, and you wouldn't want your mother to see it, don't post it!

It is also a great tool for employers to use if they have employees, that phone in sick constantly. Make sure your Facebook page from the night before doesn't reflect you having a wild night out. Taking a day off due to a hangover might be a legitimate reason for yourself to be feeling as sick as a dog, whilst barfing down the big white telephone all morning, but your boss won't be on the same page as you!! Admittedly, profiles can be blocked preventing anybody from reading it. Make sure yours is blocked if you are a wild cat!

Real Life Stories from the Experts

I had a brand new client who was leaving the next day for vacation and had NEVER had a bikini or Brazilian wax before. She came in nervous and sweaty. At the time, I was using an awful green wax (forgot the name of it). Needless to say, it clumped up in her hair and matted everything together, so I put hard wax on top of the clumped up green wax mess and it turned to a ball of glue. Scissors came out next, clumps of hair, bleeding, sweat and body odour . . . . two hours later. —Stephanie G Laynes, USA www.ssmoothskinsupply.com

A wife made an appointment for her husband's back to be waxed and he had never had a wax before. I suggested that the hair be about no more than an inch long and to try and cut it prior to the appt. This big, burly man walked into the room and was little uneasy but was ready to have the wax service. After the first rip, sweat starting rolling down is back and forehead. He asked me for a towel to hold onto cause he gets sweaty when he is nervous, so I handed him a towel and he began to bite on it and shake. After the second rip, he kept the towel in his mouth and grabbed the underside of the massage bed with both arms. After the third rip, he begged me to go to his wife to get some drugs. Needless to say, his wife was waiting with the pills in hand mumbling about him being

a FIREFIGHTER. —Stephanie G Laynes, USA www.
ssmoothskinsupply.com

The "hairy beast" was the name I gave my one client who came to see me every 2-3 months when he could afford it or the hair became so uncomfortable that he wasn't able to enjoy sex with his mate. He had hair up his shaft and sticking out of his backside. Some Esty told him to shave with a razor along his back crack and his hair was thick and bushy from the front all up and through the back. He was a two hour wax appointment just for the "boyzillian" because I had to be careful to not irritate his large haemorrhoids staring back at me. —Stephanie G Laynes, USA www.ssmoothskinsupply.com

I once had a client come into a salon that spoke very little English. He informed me that he was Russian and that he had done some research on-line about the man waxing. Throughout the service, I kept telling him that he needed to hold himself so I could wax easier around him. He kept letting go and proudly showing me his man parts. I started to get slightly angry and was just about ready to tell him to get dressed and leave my room, which in this profession we are within our rights to end a service at any time if we feel uncomfortable. I firmly told him that he needed to do this to make it easier on both of us but he didn't. So, I got out my tweezers and started to tweeze the hairs from his testes. Ouch! He soon lost his manhood and soon didn't seem to find it pleasurable anymore. I ended his service; he lay there all confused when I told him it was over. His comment was, "Huh is that it?" "Don't I get anything else?" in his stupid broken English. Not sure what website he had been looking at but he certainly wasn't getting it in my salon!! By the way, I never got a tip either . . . tight ass!! —Lesley MacArthur, USA

I came into work one morning (slightly hung-over from the night before from the staff Xmas party!). The receptionist said "Oh, you have a client on his way that is requiring a waxing from you." "What sort of waxing does he want?" I asked. "He was very vague on the phone and said he would explain it to you when he arrived." Strange! So I waited for my client who showed up larger than life all jolly and ready to go. I took him into my room and asked him what sort of wax did he want? "I really just want the bottom part doing" He tells me. "Ok, Sir, undress from the waist down and I will be back in the room shortly" I tell him. I come back in to find this rather large, heavy set gentleman on all fours on my bed with his bum cheeks spread apart! All he wanted was an anus wax! It was 8am, I was hung-over, I had just eaten a greasy breakfast and I wanted to die! —Sally Jensen, UK

A really pretty female came in for a bikini wax. She was a college, student and very chatty. I waxed around the sides of her bikini area . . . piece of cake. As I started to wax around the sides of her labia, I came across something that I had never seen before. I wasn't too sure what it was, but it resembled a cluster of blisters. It looked pretty sore, so I asked her about it. "Don't worry about it, I am pretty resilient to pain . . . it's a Herpes outbreak, that I get once a year!" WTH? Obviously, I told her I shouldn't/couldn't wax around that area as the likelihood of it spreading is very high. Thank goodness for latex gloves (that I was wearing) and get this!!!! I had to throw the whole pot of wax away as this was five or six years ago when double dipping was never known to be an issue!!! Expensive service for me that was!!!! —Sian Cooke, UK

A marine just home from his deployment was coming in for a back wax before he visited his girlfriend that he hadn't seen for nine months. He was telling me during the prepping process that he was in Afghanistan and that things were brutal, but he enjoys it and just misses his family. As I start to wax, he yelps out and nearly flies off the bed! He hated every minute of it and told me it was the most painful thing he had ever experienced! Military back packs, military boots, trudging through the hot sweltering heat and this was more painful!! Hmmmm! —Denise, USA

I was waxing a guy who flew his legs around the bed every time I tried to wax them which was pretty disturbing . . . . Or, maybe it was the fact that his lip gloss was shinier than mine . . . not sure! —Kimberly, Vancouver, Canada

Questionnaire filled out . . . all complete. Check all boxes. No Retin-A or Acutane. Perfect. Rip! Talk about lifting the skin!! Practically half her eye-lid was removed! She did confess that she took Retin-A, but was embarrassed to admit to it! She was pissed with ME!!! I told her that the paperwork told her the reasons why the questions were being asked. —Anonymous

During beauty school, my friend Tina and I decided to partner up in the eyebrow wax class. She was pretty proficient in make up application so I thought I would let her go first. One eyebrow was completed as she stood back, hands on hips proudly examining her work!! I was

very happy and hummed to myself as she started on the second one. I was going to like my new designer brows. She proceeded to wax, then stopped and gasped! There was a long period of silence. "Ms. Jay", she yelled across the room, "Come quickly." I sat upright . . . "What? What?" I asked. Ms. Jay comes over and calmly informs us that it's nothing an eyebrow pencil cannot correct. Tina had waxed my brow with a wax strip that had wax on it from the previous brow. As she placed it over my brow the wax removed a huge chunk right out of the centre of my brow!!! I was due to go on holiday to Greece for a few weeks a week later and I travelled very closely with my new eyebrow pencil!!! —Claire Barnes, USA*

We got a phone call once at the salon from a very irate mother who complained bitterly that her daughter, who was only 16, had come in to see us for a Brazilian bikini wax. My manager was off sick this day so being the head aesthetician I took the call. She was devastated that we would wax a girl that young (hey lady, it's your daughter going to the prom with other thoughts on her mind . . . saucy minx). She said she had gone to school that day very uncomfortable and with a very bad rash spreading around her voojie. I asked her what her daughter was wearing for school that day and she told me that she was wearing jeans. I told the angry mother on the phone very calmly that wearing jeans would irritate her even more and could she bring her in after school, so I could take a look at her. She agreed, but they never showed up that day or the next. I called the lady with a concerned follow-up call and she humbly apologized and told me on her way to the salon that her daughter told her she had called the wrong salon! I thought when I checked the books that there was no person with that name on there, but with divorced parent's, who knows these days, who, is called what. I do wish the angry lady would have taken it upon herself to call us back and apologize for accusing us of something we had never done!! —Jennifer, USA

I had on my books an hour-and-a half massage, (it happens once a year, the most people want around here is an hour) so I was so extremely excited, that I completely forgot, that I had just one 'little' bikini wax to do before that appointment.

I set up, lit the candles, the client came, filled out a form, then I took her to the room, showed her around and told her basically, just leave your panties on, and lay face down under the blanket . . . .

I waited a little and entered the room; she is in the bed facing down undressed. She looks up at me and said "This is just a regular bikini right?

I looked at her "Well, had you not said anything, you would have got an hour and a half massage!!"

She has been coming to me for years for bikini waxing; she even took her shirt off!!

She said "Well, I know you know what you are doing; I thought maybe there is a new way of doing it!"

We have been laughing about it ever since!

Just shows how much power you gain by earning your client's trust!

Eva Walker. Soul Escape, Esthetics Day Spa. BC. Canada

My first time at waxing a man was so different for me, because I was so used to waxing women, but I decided to focus my mind on the fact that it is no different to waxing a woman. He broke wind when I was waxing the butt crack (or earthquake is what I call this service!) He was trying to lift his butt so I could get everything down to the scrotum. The loud fart hit the air as I was about to apply the wax!!

Spa by M Melissa M, (Owner/Esthetician/MUA) Pflugerville, Texas.

Real Life Stories from Clients

I made the trek to a well-known wax studio—a place that was heavily frequented by celebrities. The owner was a bit of her celebrity herself since she worked with so many of them. Once she started on my wax, we were making small talk and she asked me how I came to find her. I told her that I heard about her on the news from a local weather girl. That sent her into a tailspin and she started telling me why this weather girl doesn't come to her anymore. The story went on for some time and she actually stopped waxing me and sat on the table next to me. If that wasn't bad enough, she took the muslin cloth that she had just ripped off of me and laid it on her thigh while she finished the story. Now I know it was my hair on the muslin but I really didn't want to look at it. She simmered down and finished. She had my flip to do the back side and when she was all done gave me a little slap on the booty. Totally creepy and totally unprofessional and I never returned.
—Cassie Piasecki, USA

I had a God-forsaken eyebrow wax with a technician who constantly kept popping gum in her mouth as she leant over me trying to wax my brows. Her gum chewing was obviously trying to mask the smell of nicotine . . . totally gross and not at all professional. No return for me! —P. Chadwick, USA

There's nothing worse than going to a salon, whether it's for hair, waxing or facials and the person working on you compares themselves to their competition down the street! Not interested . . . but the one thing I will do is try out your competition as they have to be waaaay more professional than you!! —Mary Venderbilt, USA

I was having a good day until I went for my monthly lip wax. The usual place I went to was closed for a few weeks following some severe water pipe leakage . . . so I tried some random place. As she starts to wax my lip, she steps back with her face and asks me if I had ever considered Botox for the lines around my mouth as I needed it! Hmm!!! —Sarah Mancini, USA

I went on my fantastic honeymoon with three hickies around my bikini area! They were not from a night of sex but a drastic bikini wax a few days before! It was a case of . . . . Apply the wax, stand back, and just pull it without holding me. I cried when I got home, but being the big baby that I am, I never said anything in the salon. Chicken I know! ☹ —Toni Lavacot, Orange County, California

There's nothing worse than having a technician who huffs and puffs due to their frustrations at working on my bikini hair! OK, OK, I know its super coarse . . . some have told me I am very difficult! I have now found a great gal who does an amazing job and seems to enjoy the challenge I bring to her every month! —Ruby, USA

I had a gal get wax stuck in my belly button once from my chest and stomach wax. When she got the metal plucking things out to remove it, I decided going home and taking

a shower would be safer. My wife would help me remove the big blob I am sure. —James Moore, USA

I went in for a back wax and the lady used a roller type of device. It looked like a big glue stick but had wax drip out the end. Well, she put the wax on, but it wouldn't come off. She said the wax was probably a bit too cold, so kept going over it and over it to remove it. In the end she had to pick most of it off! I felt bad for her as she was new out of school and seemed a bit upset. When I voiced my concerns nicely to the receptionist who also happened to be the manager, then that was a different story. Apparently, it was my fault as I must have had dry skin!! Ok, lady . . . . I didn't go back to your dumb place again. —Frank Parish, Vancouver, Canada

I had dark blue hard wax stuck up my nostril once! Having a stranger pick your nose was an experience I won't forget! It came out eventually with most of my brain I think! —Mike G, USA

I went to Las Vegas with the boys for a long weekend last year. So I decided I would have more chance of finding the chicks if I had my vest removed! I broke out like a teenager!! I had more pimples than I have ever had in my life!! Pretty common I heard with some waxes. I have been back a few times since as I heard your skin needs to get used to it. It did get a bit better, but not worth it. Not for me. The chicks will have to like me hairy! —Anonymous

I will tell you what I don't like when I see somebody in a salon. Drama! All some of them do is yack, yack, yack. When my eyes are closed, I am probably meditating

through the leg wax, as I admit, I find it painful! But, when you continue to yack for an hour solid about your life and your boyfriend, it makes it more painful!! Ok, I will shut up now. Thanks for allowing me to write my vent! —Marie W., London, U.K.

I was once told that I had a really nice vagina! Nice! I wasn't sure what to make of that comment, but I will keep the compliment, thank you very much! —Anonymous

I wasn't too sure why when I sometimes got a leg wax did I come out feeling stubbly. I never knew why until an esty told me it was because the paper wasn't removed correctly and I might has well have stayed home and shaved as the hair roots were still in there. Please remember girlies, I paid for a leg wax, not a shave. —Irritated in Orange County, USA

I had a bikini wax in beauty school once. I say once, because I never did it again!! They had to get the scissors out to remove the wax that was all stuck to my pubic hair. The wax felt cold and I always thought it was hot wax that is used. Not sure what went wrong and I feel bad as they are all students . . . but the teacher was on the missing list. I was sore for about a week after that. Ugh. —Phillipa Adkins, Washington, USA

I hate, hate having my feet waxed. Its part of the full leg wax . . . but the darn stuff never comes off the tops of my feet!! —Anonymous

I haven't had any really, really bad experiences. For the most part, I love visiting the salon for a wax. I am much

happier now also that most places don't double dip. I never gave it much thought before until the girl who waxes me proudly told me it was their policy. —Sarah Green, UK

Was looking forward to a leg wax with a new girl that the Salon advised I try. The whole time she waxed me, she kept complaining about how her boss was a b***h, how she never got adequate lunch breaks. I was stressed, just listening to her! Please, don't tell me your Salon politics, I have enough of my own to deal with in my own office!! —Mary Beddington. Orange County, California

It took me a while to find somebody who did an efficient bikini wax, and once when visiting L.A I came across a great place owned by a British woman. They did a great job . . . . wish they had a place in Colorado where I live! —Tina Alcala, Denver.

I was in Tenerife on holiday and decided to go to the local chemist and buy a pot of cold wax. It was a funky green colour and was applied cold. Trying to get the stuff off was a nightmare and I was left with bruises and sore patches of skin. Not to forget a sunburn as I had to walk back to the chemist with green funk still attached to my legs, to see if they had a product that I could use to remove it. All of a sudden their English wasn't too good and they acted dumb! I fumbled my way back to the hotel where I spent the next 3 hours using everything from baby oil to hot showers trying to release the stuff from my legs. The first wax I ever had was not done by a professional but by me! I eventually got it all off, minus a few sheets of skin and still hairy legs!! My next wax will certainly be done by a professional. Mary V Pinnock. Leicester. U.K

Glossary of British Terms

- Big White Telephone – toilet
- Brilliant – Awesome
- Buggers – Nuisance things
- Bum – Butt
- Cheeky – Sassy
- Crabby – Bitchy
- Crown Jewels – Penis
- Dumb as a Box of Frogs – Just plain dumb
- Ferret – Rummage around
- Jewels – Penis and testes
- Knickers – Underwear
- Lady Garden – Vagina
- Love Bite – Hickey
- Lunch Box – Penis and testes
- Mug – Face
- Shlonker – Penis
- Tacky – Sticky
- Tid-Bits – Pieces of
- Trousers – Pants
- Twigs and Berries – Penis and testes
- Verbal Diarrhoea – Overflow of mindless chatter
- Winky – Penis
- Wotsits – Your you-know-what
- Waffling – see Verbal Diarrhoea

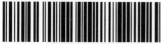
Made in the USA
Lexington, KY
30 March 2012